The
Q
Letters

The *Q* *Letters*

True Stories
of Sadomasochism

"Sir" John

Prometheus Books • Buffalo, New York

Published 1993 by Prometheus Books

97 96 95 94 93   5 4 3 2 1

Library of Congress Cataloging-in-Publication Data

John, Sir.
   The Q letters : true stories of sadomasochism / "Sir" John.
      p.   cm.
   ISBN 0-87975-821-X (cloth)
   1. Sadomasochism. I. Title.
HQ79.J64   1993
306.77′5—dc20   92-42171
                                                         CIP

Printed on acid-free paper in the United States of America.

This book is dedicated with respect, pride, thanks, and all my love to all of the wonderful women who have given themselves to me in submission.

In particular, betty, allison, sally, susan, liz, ursula, isabelle, frances, suzie, christina, sabrina, tracey, and veronica.

Contents

Foreword

As has been thoroughly and publicly documented in such books as *My Secret Garden* and many other serious books on the subject, almost everyone has secret "fantasies" that they use to add pleasure to their lives. These fantasies range from childhood dreams of being a space traveler to adult fantasies of encounters with sexual idols.

One of the most common fantasies involves what, in shorthand, is called "S/M," which stands for "Sadomasochism" or, sometimes, "Slave-Master." (The initials "B-D" are also commonly used. These stand for "Bondage and Discipline," which are frequently included in the physical manifestations of an S/M relationship.)

As *Time* magazine once reported, a "forced-sex fantasy, or something like it, is one of the most common sexual daydreams of American women." And now it appears that while many men often fantasize about taking a woman by force, many other men dream of being dominated—intellectually, physically, and even sexually—by a woman.

The words "sadism" and "masochism" are familiar to everyone; a number of books, including the classic *Story of O,* have thoroughly explored these areas. The fact that people can experience true pleasure from either giving or receiving pain—even severe pain—is generally accepted. A recent survey by *Playboy* magazine indicates that some seven percent of the U.S. population has at least experimented with S/M, and that another ten percent would like to try it.

Personal advertising columns frequently include notices from people involved in the S/M scene seeking each other. Clubs or bars exist in many major cities where "dominants" and "submissives" gather. Some of these places are outfitted with such equipment as whipping stools, suspension crosses, and the like. Even Mensa, the respected world-wide organization of people with genius-level intelligence, has organized informal "study groups" that specialize in the discussion of S/M topics.

Despite all this, for most people S/M is still only an indistinct fantasy and the idea that there are people who actually spend a part of their lives dressed in leather, or helpless in bondage, or whipping someone or being whipped, or kneeling submissively as a "slave" before a "Master" or a "Mistress," is almost unthinkable. But for perhaps as many as ten million adults in the United States alone, S/M has moved out of the world of fantasy, and into real life. For these people the symbols of leather and chains and boots and whips are no longer merely symbols but are, instead, a very important part of their lives.

John Q____ is one of these people. He has been involved in the S/M scene for more than twenty-five years. For the most part, his involvement has been quite private. Over the years John has become rather well-known inside the S/M scene. I have known him for more than ten years. But it was only two years ago that I discovered that John has kept an almost complete record of his S/M experiences, in the form of hundreds of notes, letters, diaries, photographs, and even videotape recordings. John was kind enough to allow me to go through this material; in doing so I quickly became aware of a level of commitment, imagination, and sensitivity far beyond anything else I had ever encountered in the S/M scene.

Fortunately, I was able to persuade John to arrange and edit the material for this book. I explained that I was convinced that such a book, properly done, could be very important in three ways. First, for those already in the S/M scene, it could serve as a fascinating, positive, and supportive history that could add a new dimension of insight and sensitivity and pleasure to their lives.

Second, I thought that John's experiences could demonstrate the tremendous variety of motives, activities, and relationships that exist within the S/M scene.

But most important of all, I believed that such a book could help explain to those outside the scene what S/M is *really* all about. Of all the so-called "fetishist" activities, S/M has probably the worst reputation among "straight" people . . . a reputation that ranges from "kinky" at best to outright criminal, or worse. But those of us in the scene know that in addition to providing incredibly exciting and satisfying highs—both emotional and sensual—S/M also involves understanding, honesty, sensitivity, and a tremendous amount of trust and love.

And I told John Q that I wanted "straight" people to know that.

This book is the result of those efforts. In the main, the words are John Q's, taken from his diaries and letters and memories. But also included are many letters written to John from others, mostly his submissive partners. The result is a book that presents with honesty and rare understanding a true picture of the S/M scene. It tells how people become involved in S/M; it details the nature of their relationships and activities; and it describes the fulfillments and the rewards that these S/M practitioners feel they receive from this very special part of their lives.

The material has been chosen and edited carefully to make the story of John Q and the S/M scene as honest as possible. Which brings up the most important point of all . . . and that is that this book *is* honest. It is *not* a made-up letter to the editor written to appeal to the most prurient of interests. It is *not* a product of anyone's imagination or fantasy.

Instead, John Q is a *real* person.

This is a *true* story.

And, finally, this is what S/M is *really* about.

Jim T.
Board of Directors
The Eulenspiegel Society
New York City

The Eulenspiegel Society (T.E.S.), founded in 1971, is the original association formed to allow people to freely discuss their dominant and/ or submissive fantasies, urges, and experiences. T.E.S. believes that everyone—straight, gay, or bisexual—has the right to explore and enjoy their sexual orientation without being condemned by others. T.E.S. is known and highly respected world-wide and many other similar S/M discussion groups have now been formed in almost every major city in the U.S.

Author's Note

This is a true history. It is based entirely on fact. The publisher has been given as much documentation as I could provide. I have sworn to the accuracy of those parts that could not be fully documented. As a result, I obviously cannot use the standard disclaimer about "similarity to real people" being a coincidence. It isn't. They are *very* real people. However, except where noted, I have made every effort to protect their anonymity.

J.Q.

Preface

Nothing in my early life gave me any indication that I was to become a sexual dominant. I had a normal and happy upper-middle-class upbringing. My parents loved me. I was never abused. And I never had any adolescent fantasies of that nature.

I went to an excellent prep school, graduated from Princeton, got married, served four years in the Marines, and then went to work in the advertising business.

As related in this book ("Carol"), my introduction to the S/M "scene" was completely accidental. But once I became aware of the tremendous psychological and sexual pleasures the scene made possible, I was totally hooked. I have now been involved in that scene for almost thirty years.

Many people, especially women, have asked me to explain the nature of the pleasure I get from S/M. It's hard to explain to people who have never experienced it. There is, of course, the feeling of power. That's exciting for anyone, I think. Next, I have a minor streak of sadism in my nature which, though it does not manifest itself in my regular day-to-day life, emerges when I enter the S/M scene. I take great pleasure from disciplining my submissive partners whenever I choose, placing them in various forms of bondage and then, again if I choose, tormenting them with a whip or in any number of other ways. And because I know these women have *chosen* to give me their pain and are proud and happy to give me this gift, that excitement is even more intense.

But the overriding pleasure is sexual. The bottom line is that S/M is an intense, elaborate, and incredibly exciting form of sexual foreplay. *Both* parties get sexually aroused, far beyond anything they have ever experienced. In addition, my submissive partners are available to me for absolutely any sexual activity I may choose, and they are also willing and eager participants. The result is a magnificently exciting and rewarding sexual experience . . . for *both* of us.

The root of all these pleasures is the truly submissive nature of my female partners. They have not been kidnapped. They are not coerced. They have, instead, chosen to *give* me that power and those pleasures. What an incredible gift! If you are a male reader, imagine that you are with a truly magnificent woman. She is incredibly beautiful. She is strong, intelligent, and proud of who and what she is. She is sexually experienced, inventive, and enthusiastic. You know that every other man envies you. Then imagine that you are alone with her. Without being asked or ordered, she strips herself naked, kneels at your feet, and bows her head. Then she speaks: "I give myself to you body and soul. I want you to be my Master and I beg you to allow me to be your *total* slave. I will do anything you ask. You may do to me or with me anything you want. My only desire is to serve your pleasure in absolutely any way you choose."

That may be just an exciting fantasy for many men. For me, that fantasy has come true. Many times.

For my female readers, I have learned that many, many women have secret submissive fantasies . . . not necessarily as extreme as some of those described in this book, but still involving at least sexual submission to a man. And I have also learned that many of these women are, sadly, ashamed of these fantasies, and often believe that they are the only ones who have them.

To these women I say, *you are not alone.* And, given trust and love and the right man, those fantasies can come true. And if they do, it will be tremendously exciting and rewarding, both emotionally and sexually. Indeed, a number of women have told me that experiencing S/M with me was the first time they had ever had an orgasm except by masturbation.

Finally, I want to repeat a point made by my friend, Master Jim, in the foreword. The S/M scene is *not* necessarily perverse. True, there are, unfortunately, occasional instances of outright sadism; or of people being abused against or beyond their will; or of people, both men and women, who become "slaves" only because of extremely low self-esteem and the belief that this is the only way they can get any attention at all from the opposite sex. (Or from the same sex, if that is their choice.)

I have never been involved in that kind of relationship. My submissive female partners have all been strong, proud women. They have cared for me and trusted me, and often loved me; and I have been equally proud of them, and have deeply cared for and loved them. They have chosen to submit to me of their own free will, knowing that it will give me pleasure, but knowing also that it will provide them, too, with tremendous sexual and emotional pleasure.

This type of relationship between a dominant and submissive is probably the most intense and profound possible. And when it is based on mutual pride, trust, and *love,* it is incredibly rewarding.

In short, for both parties, their dearest fantasies have come true!

Sir John Q

(I realize that this book describes a very controversial lifestyle and would welcome comments from readers—both pro and con. I would also welcome responses from those readers who are in the scene and who would like to share their own fantasies and/or experiences. Write to: John Q, 380 Bleeker Street, Box 149, New York, NY 10014.)

1

Vicky

I was twenty years old.
I was a junior in college.
I was also a virgin.

I was home on spring vacation and had a date with a new girlfriend, Vicky, a senior at a local college who was a year older than I and considerably more experienced. We had met at a Christmas party, dated three times during the winter vacation, and traded a couple of letters.

Vicky was pretty, intelligent, athletic, and enthusiastically sexy. She had quickly cut through the shyness and inferiority complex that until then had kept me from actually "making out."

On this afternoon, after playing tennis, we had gone back to Vicky's house to have supper and watch television, knowing that her parents planned to be out for the evening playing bridge. As soon as we were alone, Vicky shut off the TV and curled up next to me on the couch. Half an hour later, for the first time in my life, I found myself with a girl who was entirely naked.

By then, Vicky and I were stretched out on the floor. Vicky was lying on her back and I was kissing her breasts while, with her help and encouragement, two of my fingers had moved inside of her. Finally I took a deep breath, moved to kneel over her, and put my hands on her thighs to spread her legs.

Suddenly Vicky tensed. Her legs went rigid and she pushed against me and I heard her saying, "Oh, please, John, we can't, we can't."

Without even thinking about what I was doing, I drew back my right arm and slapped her twice across the face. "The hell we can't!" I yelled at her.

Instantly Vicky's body relaxed, her legs spread, and her hand reached out to help guide me into her. Then both her arms went around my neck and she buried her face in my shoulder.

And as I moved slowly, feeling the joy and wonder and excitement and pride of being inside a woman for the very first time, Vicky's arms pulled me tightly to her and I heard her whisper, "How did you know what I needed? How did you know?"

I didn't have the faintest idea what she was talking about.

2

Carol

I was living in New York City. I had just changed jobs, moving into
a position that involved a lot of travel, and I was in Chicago to attend
the summer furniture show. Since I represented a company that did
a lot of advertising, I was invited to a cocktail party hosted by a major
magazine. That's where I met Carol.

Carol was a typical Midwestern girl. She was tall and naturally
pretty and healthy-looking with an athletic body, long dark hair, and
a complexion that allowed her to use very little makeup. She was also
very friendly and easy to relate to and for two hours we stood in a
corner, talking. I learned that Carol was twenty-four years old and a
junior copywriter for a small Chicago advertising agency.

I soon decided that I wanted to spend more time with her, preferably
in a quieter place, and so I finally suggested that we leave the party
and go somewhere for steaks and beers. Carol accepted the invitation,
suggesting a small dark restaurant somewhere off Rush Street.

Soon after we arrived at the restaurant, however, things sort of
fell apart, and after a couple more drinks Carol's friendliness turned
to something approaching bitchiness—not directed at me personally,
but at men in general.

"There aren't any real men any more," she told me. "All the men
I know are weaklings and babies. I can beat them in swimming and

I can beat them at tennis. And they're all such assholes! I mean, all I have to do is wiggle my little finger and they fall all over themselves to do anything I want."

"They're all just so stupid," she continued, "and they're all lousy in bed, too. They're like little boys and it's like they're all afraid of me and they don't know what the hell they're doing. And worst of all, they always ask me if they were any good. For Christ's sake! They're too stupid to even know when a girl has an orgasm! And besides," Carol went on, "if they were really men they wouldn't worry so goddamn much. They'd just take me and fuck me and that would be so great; but instead they just mince around and damn near beg me to let them go to bed with me, and it makes me so mad I usually just tell them to fuck off!"

This went on all during dinner and by the time we finished, I'd had it up to my ears. I'd lost all interest in doing anything except getting rid of Carol as quickly as possible. I'd spent enough of my life feeling insecure with women and I didn't need to go back to that again.

So after dinner I walked Carol to the parking lot where she had left her car, shook hands with her, and figured that was that.

I was wrong.

Three days later, on a Saturday morning, the phone in my hotel room rang while I was shaving. It was Carol wanting to know if I'd like to come out to her family's home in Glencoe the next day for cocktails and Sunday dinner. Since I'd spent five straight days eating in restaurants or my hotel room, a home-cooked meal sounded pretty good. Besides, I figured that with her family around it ought to be a lot more pleasant than the first meeting, so I accepted.

Carol gave me directions, and the next day I rented a car. About five o'clock in the afternoon I arrived at Carol's home in Glencoe, a lovely upper-class suburb right on the lake, about twenty-five miles north of Chicago. Carol's house turned out to be a beautiful home in what seemed to be the best part of town. It was a big three-story Tudor-style house set well back from the street on a large, tree-covered lot. There was a curved driveway that went past the house to a paved turn-around area, in front of a two-car garage that was connected to the rear of the house by a breezeway.

Parking the car next to the house, I walked around to the front where I was greeted by Carol. She gave me a smile, a big hello and a quick kiss, and then led me inside. And the first thing she said was,

"I hope you like my cooking. Mom and Dad are up at our summer place for two weeks."

Carol was wearing a low-cut sundress that showed off both her tan and her body, and suddenly it wasn't too hard to forget about our first meeting. And when she made me a gin and tonic, sat cross-legged on the floor in front of me, and asked me all about my job, I decided that she had just been in a bad mood that first night.

After an hour or so, Carol made me a fresh drink, excused herself, and headed toward the kitchen. Assuming she was going to start dinner, I stayed where I was and began looking through the Sunday paper that was on the table. I wasn't really paying attention to the time, but finally it seemed that quite a while had gone by, so I went out to the kitchen to see if there was anything I could do to help.

Carol wasn't in the kitchen.

I checked the breakfast room and dining room and went out the back door to the patio but I didn't find her. Finally I called her name.

"I'm down here," I heard her answer.

"Where's 'here'?" I called back.

"Down in the rec room."

"Where's that?"

"The door next to the refrigerator."

I opened the door and went down a flight of stairs to a large pine-panelled room. There was a pool table, a beautiful bar, a fireplace, and a group of chairs around a television set.

And there was Carol, standing in the middle of the room with her hands held high over her head, completely naked!

I didn't really believe it at first and I froze at the bottom of the stairs. That's when Carol began talking. I couldn't believe what she was saying, either. She was rambling and loud—on the edge of hysteria, it seemed. I didn't understand everything Carol said, but what I could make out was pretty wild.

"Please don't be mad but this is the only way I could think of that I wouldn't be able to boss a man around and I've never done this before but my parents won't be home for two weeks and you can do anything you want to me. You can rape me or you could whip me to death even, and the neighbors couldn't hear and I can't get loose and the keys to the handcuffs are on the bar and I put a riding crop there, too, and I'm really helpless. I've never done this before with anyone, but I thought about it and how this would be the only way I could let a man be a man and there isn't anything I can do to stop you from doing anything you want to me, and . . ."

By then Carol was repeating herself, but I had picked up on the word "handcuffs." Finally I pulled myself together and walked over to her. She really was handcuffed—one cuff on each wrist with the connecting chain padlocked to another chain that was, in turn, padlocked to a pipe that ran across the ceiling.

It's hard to explain what I felt. I'm not sure I understood it myself. First, I was shocked. I was also scared. Then I wanted to laugh at her, but somehow I couldn't. And combined with all these feelings was the fact that I just didn't really believe any of it was happening.

Mainly, I didn't believe that Carol actually couldn't get loose if she really wanted to, so the first thing I did, dumb as it sounds, was tickle her. Her reactions quickly proved that she really was helpless.

That's when I got mad!

I think that I finally understood the age-old complaint of so many women who are angered by men who, "don't care anything about me as a person . . . they just look at me as a body." That's the way I felt. Sort of "used," I think the expression is. In addition, I couldn't quite buy her claim about not having ever done this before. Considering the chains, the locks, the handcuffs, and the riding crop, it seemed pretty clear to me that Carol was an old hand at this game and that she had played it with many other men who, based on her bitching about all men being pushovers, had undoubtedly gone along obediently with what I then considered her "sick" ideas about fun.

But not me. I was going to teach her a lesson! I wasn't going to whip her, of course. That would make me sick, too. But I sure as hell could scare the shit out of her!

"You're sick!" I yelled at her. "And as far as I'm concerned I wouldn't touch you with a ten-foot pole! And if you really can't get loose, you damn well better hope somebody comes home before you starve to death, because I'm going to leave you right where you are, and I don't give a shit what you do or what happens to you!" And then I stamped back up the stairs to the kitchen and slammed the door.

My plan was to leave her there long enough to really scare her. But then I decided that she wouldn't really believe I meant it if she didn't hear me leave the house, so I went to the front door, fixed the lock so that I could get back in, and left, slamming the door behind me as hard as I could.

Even better, I thought next, would be to let her hear the car drive away, so I went to it, started it up, raced the engine loudly, and pulled out of the driveway, intending to drive around the block a few times before going back.

It didn't work out that way. The more I thought about it, the more intrigued I got with my own "game" and, yes, excited, too. And the farther I got into it, the more exciting it got!

So I didn't drive around the block. Instead I drove back to downtown Chicago where, an hour later, I was sitting at a table in the famous Pump Room, sipping a cocktail and studying the menu.

I don't think I've ever eaten so slowly in my life. I even chewed slowly. I took extra time deciding about dessert, and then I had two Drambuies and a couple of extra cups of coffee. And all the time I sat there, the excitement grew and grew, together with a feeling that I had never had before—the thrill of knowing that I had total power over another human being. Twenty or thirty miles away in the basement of a house was a beautiful naked woman in chains and totally helpless. She could struggle and she could scream and she could even pray, but there was only one person in the world who could help her and that person was me.

I thought about how long she would stay there . . . how long her "punishment" would last. I thought about how she had looked, standing there with her arms over her head pulling her breasts high, and about how maybe I should have turned the lights off so that she would have been left chained there alone in the darkness. I thought about how she must be feeling by now . . . helpless, exhausted, and terrified.

I ordered another Drambuie, sat there, and let the excitement build.

It was almost ten o'clock by the time I left the Pump Room and nearly eleven when I coasted into the driveway of Carol's house with the car headlights off. It had been more than six hours since I'd left and I wanted to make sure that someone hadn't come home, let Carol go, and was waiting for me. Leaving the car at the end of the driveway, I walked across the lawn to the house and looked in the windows of the living room and kitchen. I saw no one. The front door was unlocked as I had left it; I let myself in as quietly as possible and stood in the front hall a few minutes. There was no sign of anyone being home.

I took my shoes off, tiptoed to the kitchen, and carefully opened the door at the top of the stairs leading down to the rec room. At first I couldn't hear anything, but after a while I heard a sort of whimper and then the sound of the chain scraping on the pipe and, finally, Carol's voice, low and hoarse and exhausted, saying, "Oh, God, please, please, please, please, please, please, please . . . ," and then the whimpering sound again.

I went all the way down the steps where I saw Carol half-hanging by her arms, her head bent forward with her hair, tangled and damp with sweat, partly covering her face. I stood there watching her for maybe three minutes before she finally lifted her head and saw me.

She jumped and let out a little scream, and then she put her head down again and began to cry, and while she was crying she kept repeating, "Oh thank God! Thank God! Thank God!" over and over again.

I walked over to her. She was shaking and crying. Her wrists were both raw, and there was dried blood on one of them. I put my hand under her chin and lifted her head. "Look at me," I ordered her. She opened her eyes and sniffled. "Say something," I said.

Little by little Carol got control of herself, and finally she was able to talk to me. She told me how at first she was sure that I was kidding and figured I'd be back in a few minutes. After a while—she didn't know how long—she became angry because I was taking so long. But finally she began to think that maybe I really wasn't ever coming back, and she became terrified.

"I screamed and screamed," Carol told me, beginning to cry again, "and that's when I cut my wrists, jerking on the handcuffs. I don't know how long I did that. It was awful." She dropped her head and began sobbing again. I stood there watching her; when she had calmed down, I lifted her head again.

"Go on," I said.

Carol told me that she finally had given up and had just stood there crying and praying. She said she thought she had partly fainted a couple of times but that the pain in her wrists brought her back each time the weight of her body pulled on them. Finally she had become sort of numb and had gone into something like a trance. After that she didn't remember much of anything until she suddenly saw me standing at the bottom of the stairs. She didn't have any idea how long she had been that way.

By this time Carol had stopped crying and seemed to have control of herself. "What do you want now?" I asked her.

Carol looked at me for a long time and then she slowly bowed her head. "That's up to you," she said. "You can do anything you want."

I whipped her.

I didn't use the riding crop. Instead, I took off my belt and wrapped it around my right hand a couple of times, leaving about two feet free, and I whipped her with that. I started on her back, lightly at first, and then a little harder, and then harder still while her back slowly became covered with the red marks my belt left on her skin. Each time I hit Carol, her head jerked back, her body flinched, and she made a sort of low growling sound halfway between a scream and a sigh.

After a while I moved to her ass and the backs of her legs, but finally I stopped and walked around in front of her. Carol's eyes were closed and she was panting. When I whipped her once hard across the belly, she cried out, opened her eyes, and looked at me.

"Do you like getting whipped?" I asked her.

She shook her head. "No," she whispered.

"Then why don't you ask me to stop?"

Carol looked me right in the eye for a few seconds, and then she answered. "Because you can do anything you want to me."

I cannot possibly describe the feeling that went through me when I heard those words. Power, excitement, sex, and so many other things all combined into one almost electric shock of sensation. I reached out with both hands and stroked her breasts for a minute while Carol stood there quietly, staring at me. Then, without warning, I took each of her nipples between a thumb and forefinger and pinched them both at once until she screamed. Then I took my belt and started whipping her again, this time on her belly and across her breasts as well as her back.

I don't know how long it went on . . . how many times my belt bit into her taut and extended body . . . but after a while, Carol started screaming for real and finally I heard her voice begging me to stop.

"Look at me," I ordered her. She picked up her head and opened her eyes. Her face was covered with tears. "What did you say?" I asked.

"Oh, please stop," she begged, crying. "Please stop whipping me. Please, please, please, please!" She dropped her head again.

Very slowly I whipped her fifteen more times: five across her back, five across her belly, and, finally, five across her breasts, swinging hard. Each time my belt hit her, she screamed and in between the lashes she kept repeating, "Oh, please, no . . . please, no . . . please, no . . . please, no."

After those fifteen final lashes, I dropped the belt and stripped off my clothes. I went to the bar, got the keys, and I unlocked the chain, leaving the handcuffs on Carol's wrists. I pulled her down onto the floor and held her hands over her head with one hand, using the chain between the cuffs to hold her there. Then, using my other hand to balance myself, I drove into her as hard as I could, slamming my body against hers while she began to scream again.

I lasted maybe thirty seconds before exploding inside her.

Carol stayed on the floor, lying unmoving on her back with her hands still over her head, crying quietly while I dressed and left. I didn't say anything. I didn't even look at her. I just walked up the stairs and out of the house, got into my car, and drove back to Chicago.

I slept late the next morning. By the time I woke up, the feeling of power and excitement had gone and had been replaced by acute guilt which, as I relived the previous evening, grew worse and worse. I called myself every name I could think of—"filthy," "animal," "kinky," "pervert," "sick," "dirty" . . . on and on. I thought about calling Carol but I didn't have the nerve. I couldn't do it, just as I couldn't accept what I'd done. All my life I had believed that that kind of behavior was psychotic, and I was totally disgusted with myself.

The next day, on the flight back to New York, it was still the same, and that night when my wife tried to welcome me home by making love to me, I just curled myself into a ball and told her I wasn't feeling well. It was the truth. It went on that way for at least two months, but one morning I woke up feeling hornier than I had for weeks. I woke my wife and made love to her but as I was about to come, I suddenly remembered that just before waking up I had been dreaming about whipping Carol.

That broke it for me. I dreamed about whipping Carol again, except in this dream Carol turned into my wife. A few days later, while making love to my wife, I found myself fantasizing about *her* being tied up.

Not long after that, I was reading a paperback novel that included a description of a girl being beaten. This time, instead of turning off I got turned on, and so I went and found a copy of Mickey Spillane's *Vengeance Is Mine,* which ends with a vivid description of Mike Hammer's girlfriend, Velda, hanging naked by her wrists and being whipped by "the guy in the pork pie hat." I had read this book years before without any particular feeling at the time, but now it was exciting to me and I read that ending over and over.

Eventually I had it all sorted out. There was nothing unnatural about being excited about what had happened with Carol. Instead, it would have been unnatural if I *hadn't* been turned on. After all, I was with a beautiful woman who was naked, helpless, and begging me to do anything I wanted with her. Any normal man would have reacted the same way, so there was nothing to feel guilty about.

What I didn't realize just then was how very important it would all become to me.

●　●　●

The following March, I happened to see Carol's picture in the Sunday edition of *The New York Times*. She had become engaged to a young lawyer whose family lived on Long Island, and a June wedding was planned.

I thought briefly about sending them a riding crop as a wedding present, but decided against it.

3

My Wife

I never told my wife about Carol.

But once I had gotten my own head squared away, I immediately decided that if I was going to be "into" S/M, the one person I really wanted to share it with was my wife.

I found a couple of books—either novels that included some not-too-rough S/M activities or other "sex technique" books with references to the extra sexual excitement that couples could get from at least playful bondage games. There wasn't much being written about the subject back then, so it took a while to find the kind of books I was looking for.

I gave them to my wife to read but got no reaction either way.

Finally I asked my wife what she thought. In the simplest terms, she said that, although the idea didn't turn her on particularly, she was game to try.

So finally, one night, I tied my wife to the bed and teased her sexually for a long time before making love to her. Afterwards she commented that it was uncomfortable.

On another night, I talked my wife into tying me up and playing with me, but that didn't work because I had to keep suggesting things for her to do.

It ended abruptly two weeks later, when I tied my wife up again, made love to her until she had an orgasm, and then took my belt and told her I'd like to whip her lightly to see if it was exciting. She didn't say anything, but she did close her eyes and nod her head.

I whipped her very lightly twice across her lower legs. Then twice across her thighs and twice, still very lightly, across her belly. And then I whipped her once across her right breast.

She jumped, opened her eyes, and looked at me. "We'd better stop this right now," she said.

We never tried it again.

But the need in me was still there and still growing. Before long I started out alone on a long and fascinating search for fulfillment.

4

The Learning Begins

During the four or five years after Carol, I went through a stage of ever-increasing involvement in the world of S/M. It was something like the average teenager goes through in his initial involvement in sex. There was a lot of experimentation, a lot of false starts, a lot of variety, and, most of all, a lot of excitement.

Also a lot of lessons learned. Lessons about how to find submissive partners or, better yet, how to develop them. Lessons about the infinite variety of types of submissive females—and males—and the equally infinite variety of degrees of submission. And, finally, the same lessons about the varieties and degrees of involvement among dominants.

Most important of all, lessons about where in all that variety *I* fit in . . . exactly what kind of dominant I was going to be and what kind of submissive partners would provide the fulfillment my new dominant personality required and, indeed, *deserved.* The following excerpt from a letter I wrote to a submissive explains the differences:

. . . Since we haven't met, it is difficult for me to predict with any accuracy exactly what kind of activities we might get into if we were to actually meet. One reason is that so far, at least, your two letters haven't given me any real clues as to what kind of a submissive you might turn out to be. (As a matter of fact, since you say you have

never been with any "real" Masters, you may not even know yourself.

But maybe the following will help you place yourself.

First, there is the "Classic Masochist"—the person who gets fulfillment from pain. For the true masochist, this fulfillment is sexual—pain is a turn-on—an alternative form of sexual foreplay or, in some cases, not even foreplay. Instead, the pain by itself leads to the actual achievement of orgasm. Sometimes masochists aren't really submissive, at least not intellectually. They don't consider themselves "slaves." They just really enjoy pain, at least up to a certain level, and in some cases this level can be pretty extreme.

But there is also what I call the "Psychological Masochist." This type gets fulfillment from pain, too, but in these cases the fulfillment is emotional rather than sexual. In short, for whatever real or imagined reasons, these people feel that they deserve to be punished. They feel guilty and they need pain to relieve this guilt. In frequent cases they go out of their way to provoke their dominant partners, deliberately doing something that they will be punished for, even though, in their minds, the punishment is in atonement for their hidden guilt, not the overt act of provocation. (By the way, this type of submissive doesn't appeal to me very much.)

Then there's the "Classic O" type* *. . . the submissive who accepts submission as a gift of love to her Master. She does not enjoy pain—she screams when she is whipped—but she knows that her Master derives pleasure from her pain and humiliation, and because she loves him, she offers him these gifts of her suffering. And despite the fact that she hates the pain, she often begs her Master/lover to be more and more cruel, because in her mind the greater the pain the greater her gift and, therefore, the greater her expression of love.*

Next, there is a rather interesting and frequently exciting type of submissive whom I will call the "Challenger." In reality she may not really be submissive at all, but still she seeks out relationships with dominant men and then, in effect, "challenges" them to dominate her. She constantly "rebels" to test their commitment to the dominant role. Frequently she will find that the so-called dominant isn't strong enough to handle her, and either he will chicken out or she will drop him. But when such a submissive runs into a really strong "Master," one determined to dominate her and strong-willed enough to carry through

---

*After "O," the submissive heroine of the classic S/M novel, *The Story of O.*

on that determination, the "challenger" shifts to a test of both their limits. If her Master has given her one hundred lashes, she will ask for one hundred and fifty the next time, and she will glory in her ability to continually challenge both his ability to impose his domination upon her and her ability to endure it.

Finally, there is one other type who is hard to put a label on, but I'll call her the "Classic Submissive." This person is a sort of emotional offshoot of the "Classic Masochist." This person derives, indeed requires, both the psychological and sexual pleasure and fulfillment that she can find only through the act of "total submission" to her chosen "Master." It's not just pain, although her Master does whip her. It's not just any one thing at all. Instead it is the fulfillment achieved by the total giving over of her mind and her body and her will to a Master who is, in turn, equally total in his ability to dominate every aspect of their relationship. In a way, this sounds a lot like "O," but the difference is that while "O" submits to prove her love to her Master, the "Classic Submissive" submits for the fulfillment of her own personal need to be submissive. And despite the totality of the domination and submission, it is usually a relationship also based on total and mutual trust and love. For me, this is the best S/M relationship of all.

That letter was actually written several years later. There was no way I could have written it in back in the beginning for the simple reason that I didn't know about all these things or people then.

But I was learning, and over the next few years I met all of them.

5

Paula
("Classic Masochist")

Advertisement

Young attractive female with vixenish tendencies seeks a male tiger who can take me to his lair and tame me. I will fight and claw but the right man will teach me to obey. Only those strong-willed enough to impose their desires by force on a willful woman should answer.

Years ago, about the only publication that carried this kind of advertising was a tabloid called *Confidential Flash,* which was published in Canada and sold semi-under-the-counter at newsstands in places like Times Square. "Adult bookstores" hadn't really been established yet, and magazines and newspapers like *Screw* and *Corporal* were still years away.

The advertisements themselves were considerably less direct than they are now. Words like "cock" and "fuck," and even "bondage" or "S/M," were not permitted. Instead, code words were used, such as "Greek Culture" (anal sex), "French" (oral sex), "Roman Culture" (orgies), "Polaroid Sessions" (nudism), "English Training" (discipline), and so on.

But despite this, the messages came through with reasonable clarity, as in the advertisement quoted above, the first one I ever answered. My letter was equally subtle and, after describing myself physically, I assured my new pen pal that I was indeed a truly dominant male looking for a woman whom I could "train."

Back came my first letter from a prospective submissive. This time it was hardly subtle.

Dear Sir John,

Thank you for your letter. If it is honest and you are sincere, you may be the man I've been looking for.

I am 28 years old, five foot seven, and attractive with long reddish brown hair, a good body, and "vixenish" eyes, with a personality to match.

I am a female tiger and many men have tried to tame me and make me a kitten but not many have succeeded. Those few who have are the ones who were masterful enough to force me into bondage and then make me endure the touch of Sir Nine-Tails. In addition, they have explored my body's openings with various implements and ultimately tamed me and trained me to kneel before them in submission and acknowledge their mastery.

Perhaps you are strong enough to tether me to your whipping post and impose upon me the discipline and humiliation that will ultimately subdue me, but it will not be easy. If you would like to try, write to me again and let us see where it leads.

Paula O

I wrote, of course, and Paula wrote back again, and after still one more exchange of letters we wound up talking on the telephone. Paula on the phone was something else . . . somewhat coarser, a Bronx accent, and considerably more direct.

"I don't suppose you have a soundproof dungeon?" I remember her asking.

"No."

"Too bad," she said. "I love to scream. Some day some of you Masters are going to get together and build a soundproof cabin out in the woods somewhere so that your subjects can scream all they want to."

"Have you ever done that?" I asked.

"Just once," Paula told me. "Some guy took me out in the woods.

I think it was Cape Cod or someplace like that, and it was after the season, and he tied me between two trees and I screamed and screamed."

"Do you like getting whipped?"

"No, but that's the only way you'll be able to fuck me. Most guys just want to fuck and I hate that, so I fight and fight and I only fuck the ones who beat me into it."

I never could resist a challenge.

I finally met Paula in a bar on 86th Street in New York, near an apartment I'd borrowed from a friend for the evening. She was a tall, leggy girl with a nice slender body. She was quite pretty despite the extremely exaggerated makeup, particularly around the eyes.

In person, Paula was not nearly as self-assured as she had been on the phone. Instead, she was quiet—almost hesitant—but after two drinks and some small talk, she readily agreed to go back to the apartment with me.

That afternoon, in preparation for my meeting with Paula, I had acquired my first "official" S/M paraphernalia. In a novelty shop near Times Square I had purchased two pairs of handcuffs, and at Uncle Sam's Umbrella Shop (the forerunner of such stores as The Pleasure Chest) I had bought my very first whip—a nicely braided cat-o'-nine-tails made of soft but sturdy leather.

As soon as I closed the door of the apartment behind us, I took Paula's wrists and handcuffed them behind her. She offered no resistance at all. Instead she became almost motionless, staring at me with wide eyes . . . not exactly frightened but definitely watchful. She was wearing slacks, which I quickly stripped from her along with her shoes, garter belt, stockings, and panties. I put the second pair of handcuffs on her ankles. Then I freed one of her wrists and stripped her the rest of the way, removing her sweater, blouse, and bra.

Paula was naked now, but still she showed no resistance, so I took a piece of clothesline, tied it to the handcuff still on her left wrist, and tied her arm to the top hinge of the front hall closet door. Then I took the other pair of handcuffs from her ankles and in the same way tied her right arm to the top hinge of the kitchen door, which was on the other side of the fairly wide hallway. I finished by using more clothesline to tie Paula's ankles to the lower hinges of the same two doors, leaving her spread-eagled there in the hallway, arms pulled high and wide and legs spread apart.

All through these preparations there had been no resistance or reaction from Paula, and I was tempted to congratulate myself for being so overwhelmingly dominant that she didn't dare put up a fight. It turned out that this was hardly the case.

I took my new whip and started on her ass—quite slowly at first, and not too hard. Still no reaction from Paula. She barely flinched.

I moved up to her back and began making the lashes harder. Still nothing. I swung the whip harder still. Nothing. Very hard. No reaction at all.

"I thought you liked to scream," I said.

Paula turned her head to look at me over her shoulder. Then she wiggled her ass a little and grinned at me. "I thought you were going to whip me," she said.

I turned loose and literally flogged her, using the heavy whip across her legs and ass and back and shoulders, swinging almost as hard as I could. Finally, Paula began making a kind of low, steady whining sound.

I moved around so I could whip the front of her body, and now the whip fell across her belly and then her breasts, which quickly became covered with the marks left by the nine braided leather lashes. Paula's head was thrown back. Her eyes were closed and her knees were bent so that she was partially hanging from the handcuffs on her wrists. It seemed as if she were deliberately arching her back to make her breasts more vulnerable, even leaning her body into the whip as it curled into her.

By then Paula was moaning steadily, the sound punctuated by a kind of harsh "hah!" each time the heavy whip slammed into her. But she never screamed.

I quit before she did. I had stripped to the waist and was drenched with sweat, as was Paula. Her entire body from her knees to her neck was covered with the marks of the whip and although there was no blood, there were several places where the skin had been broken. When Paula realized that I had stopped, she opened her eyes and looked at me.

"I think you've had enough," I said, and I began untying her, freeing her ankles first and then her wrists. When her arms were free, Paula put them around my neck and sort of hung on me, and I realized that she was a little weak; but after a minute or two she straightened up, hugged me, and stepped back. There was a full-length mirror on the back of the closet door, which Paula used to inspect her body.

"Nice," she said at last.

"I've never whipped anyone like that," I told her.

"You did pretty good for the first time," Paula told me.

"You didn't scream."

"Wrong king of whip," Paula advised. It seems my new whip with its nine braided lashes spread the impact over a wide area, and while it hurt, it didn't cause the sharp, concentrated "cutting" pain that a single-stranded whip delivers.

"You mean blood?"

"Sure, sometimes. That's when I really start screaming. But you did OK. It was nice."

She smiled at me. "You want to fuck now?"

I passed.

6

Nancy
("Classic Submissive")

My first meeting with Nancy was somewhat out of the ordinary. I was at a Christmas cocktail party at the old London Terrace apartment complex on West 23rd Street in New York. It was a large 3-bedroom apartment shared by three guys I didn't know. I had been invited at the last minute by a friend of one of the hosts, and he and his date were the only two people at the party that I had ever met.

I spent the usual time sipping a drink and exchanging "where do you live" and "where do you work" small talk with various people while I quietly appraised the various single ladies. Before too long it became clear that most of the guests had come as couples and that the three or four women who had come alone had already paired up, so about nine o'clock I decided to leave. But before going I asked one of the hosts to point me toward a bathroom.

"End of the hall," he told me, pointing, but when I got there there were two doors, both closed. I opened the wrong one.

It was a bedroom. In the middle of the king-size bed lay a pretty dark-haired girl on her side, reading a magazine. She had a sheet pulled up to her waist but as much as I could see of her was entirely naked.

I stopped short and started to close the door again, but before I could the girl looked up and smiled at me.

"Hi."

"Who are you?" she asked.

"I'm John."

"I'm Nancy." Since she had given me no indication that she was at all embarrassed, I decided to keep talking.

"Do you live here?" I asked.

"Oh, no. I date the guys."

I wasn't sure I'd heard the plural. "The *guys?*"

"Yes. The three guys who live here."

"Which one are you with tonight?" I asked.

Nancy rolled over onto her back, stretched her arms high over her head for a minute, and then sat up, pulling a couple of pillows behind her. She looked at me for a minute and then grinned. "I'm with all of them," she said.

I didn't say anything.

"I'm greedy," she continued. "I made love with Charlie about an hour ago and now I'm waiting to see who takes the next turn."

"That's a pretty interesting arrangement," I commented.

"It's a neat arrangement," Nancy said. "I love to fuck."

That seemed like a good line to leave on. Besides I couldn't think of anything to say. So I just nodded my head, closed the door, and left.

But I'd already made up my mind that some way or other I was going to see Nancy again.

It took me six weeks.

My first date with Nancy was a surprise. What I expected—at least what I was looking for—were a few hours with a good-looking lady who would be fun to be with and and great in bed. I got all of that, but so much more.

Nancy was, and still is, one of the brightest women I have ever known. We met after work at the old Ad Lib bar on Madison Avenue and eventually went on to eat at P. J. Clarke's over on Third. By ten o'clock we were still there and still talking, having covered everything from the new, hot movies to the latest fashions.

I'd learned that Nancy was twenty-six years old, had gone to Wellesley, and had a masters degree in English from Columbia. Her family lived in New Jersey but she had her own apartment on Barrow Street in the Village. In addition to being well-educated, Nancy was well-read, and with a job as a researcher for a major news magazine she knew more about what was going on in the world than most people. As I told her later, I would have thoroughly enjoyed spending an evening with her whether we went to bed or not.

But we did go to bed, at her apartment, and she proved to be just as uninhibited at making love as she was doing everything else. She was the first girl I'd ever slept with who made it totally obvious that she enjoyed sex as much as I did, and it was just plain great for both of us.

Afterward, we lay in bed and started talking again. I told Nancy that I'd often had fantasies about meeting a girl as enthusiastic about making love as she was. And that's when things took a sudden and interesting turn.

She started kidding me about my fantasies and I asked her about hers. After a while we got sort of serious and I found myself telling her about Carol in Chicago. As I talked, Nancy grew very quiet. By the time I got to the part about coming back to Carol's house after having left her chained up and alone for several hours, Nancy was lying perfectly still with her eyes closed. She reached out to hold onto my hand and then squeezed it tightly.

Although I decided to leave out the details, I did tell Nancy that I had whipped Carol before making love to her, and then I told her about how I had felt so guilty afterward but had finally gotten over it. After I'd finished the story, I lay there next to Nancy. Neither of us said anything for a while, but finally Nancy took a deep breath and whispered, "Oh, God!"

I wasn't sure whether that meant Nancy was turned on or turned off, so I didn't say anything. But then she rolled over, put her arm around my neck, hugged herself against me, and started talking in a low steady whisper.

She was definitely turned on!

She talked for a long time. I had touched on a fantasy that she had had since she was a little girl but, despite her total lack of inhibitions about everything else, this was something that she'd never had the nerve to talk about to anyone, let alone actually explore.

"I've never gone so far as having fantasies about actually being whipped," Nancy told me, "and I'm not sure I could handle that, but the idea of being tied up—of being completely helpless with a man so that he could do absolutely anything to me sexually, I've dreamed of that. And I've dreamed about being raped, too, ever since I was a teenager, but I really thought I was the only one, and that nobody else ever felt that way. I knew long ago that I was different from my girlfriends in the way I really loved sex and didn't feel guilty about it the way so many of them do. But ever since I was maybe ten or twelve, I've had those fantasies and it's the one thing I've never been able to talk to anyone about."

Until me.

Her fantasy came true that night. From a bondage standpoint it was hardly classy. Nancy didn't have any rope, so I wound up using my necktie, two scarves, and an electrical extension cord which I padded with a handkerchief. I tied her spread-eagled on her bed, lying on her back, and I used one more scarf to blindfold her.

I turned on the radio, found some quiet music, and then pulled a chair up next to the bed and just sat there quietly, watching her. It was fascinating. At first Nancy lay perfectly still, breathing very slowly. But as the minutes went by, she began breathing more quickly, taking fast shallow little breaths, almost as if she'd been exercising. And every once in a while she would suddenly tense, as if she were flinching, and she'd suck her belly in tight for a second before relaxing again.

Her nipples were as hard as pebbles, standing up from her breasts. Finally she opened her mouth slightly, her breathing changing almost to a pant. She began pulling a little on her bonds while her hips moved very slowly, as if she were making love.

After maybe ten minutes or more, the waiting got to her. "You son of a bitch!" she muttered. It was almost as if she were talking to herself.

I didn't answer her. I just sat there and watched her, still not touching her and not making a sound while Nancy continued her gentle squirming. Finally I reached out and used just the tip of one finger to touch her very softly on the nipple nearer to me. Nancy jumped violently and screamed. She started straining hard against her bonds, trying, it seemed, to arch her back as if begging me to touch her again.

I left her alone again for another few minutes, and then I gently touched the other nipple. Another jump and another scream.

Then I began for real.

I started by using just the tip of one finger to touch her just as lightly as I possibly could, and I traced slowly over the entire length of her body, from behind her ear, across her face, down her neck to her shoulder, slowly up the side of her breast and across the nipple, and then down across her ribs and belly slowly, slowly, as Nancy raised her hips to meet my finger. But at the last minute I moved it to the side so that it traced down the inside of her thigh and lower leg and finally across the bottom of her foot. Then it moved back upward, along the outside of her leg and hip and waist and upper body until it was back to where it had started. And then I did the same thing on the other side and then back to the near side again—slowly up and down her body, over and over again.

Nancy was twisting her body as much as her restraints would allow, and each time my finger got close to her cunt she would try to lift and move her hips in an effort to make my finger go where she so desperately wanted it to go, but she never succeeded.

Bathed in sweat, Nancy finally began to make a low-pitched steady whining sound and after a long time she began to beg, "Oh, please . . . please . . . please . . . please . . . please . . . please!"

At last I ended the teasing and paused to study her. God, she was so beautiful! Her body was slowly twisting and the muscles in her flat belly kept clenching and unclenching while her breath came in short raw gasps as she repeated, "please . . . please . . . please . . . please!"

I moved to kneel between her legs and put my hands on her, moving them firmly and slowly up over her belly to her breasts, which I cupped gently at first and then harder until I suddenly pinched both her nipples quickly but very hard so that Nancy screamed, but I had already let them go. I leaned forward and gently kissed both nipples and then my tongue began tracing the same path that my fingers had before, but this time when she raised her hips I let my tongue find her clitoris.

Almost immediately Nancy screamed again, but this time it wasn't caused by frustration or pain but by her orgasm.

She kept right on screaming through two more orgasms and then, while she was still screaming, I reached back to untie her ankles, put her legs up over my shoulders, and drove into her with my cock.

Nancy climaxed one more time before I did, but it was close.

Over the next several months I helped Nancy explore her fantasy. We slowly progressed to longer and longer sessions of her submission to total helplessness and prolonged sensual "torture," and always I would make her beg for release. Finally one evening, instead of begging me to allow her an orgasm, Nancy begged me to whip her, and so I took my belt and after I was inside her I began whipping her breasts and belly, slowly and lightly at first, but then faster and harder.

And then, instead of, "please, please, please, please," I heard Nancy whispering, "Yes, yes, yes, yes, yes, YES!"

It lasted for seven months, and each time we were together it was more intense than the last. We kept trying new things—usually things that I'd read or heard about, but sometimes things that Nancy wanted to try. It was Nancy who wanted to see if she could handle being actually suspended, so one night I hung her by her wrists, whipped her, and brought her to orgasm with a vibrator before taking her down. Later she was also hung by her ankles.

Nancy bought several different whips and asked me to use them so that she could see what they felt like, and she was also the one who one night brought home some clothespins, announcing, "Tonight I want to find out what it's like to have my nipples tortured." It seems that she'd been reading, too.

And more than once, when I was ready to stop, Nancy would ask me to continue whatever torment—physical or sexual—that I was inflicting on her. "Just a little more, John," she'd beg. "I want to find out how much I can take."

We never found out what her limits were. I was married and Nancy was still dating one of the three guys from the apartment where we had met. One night she showed up wearing an engagement ring. "It's our last date," she said. "I'm going to marry Charlie." She looked down at her ring and then back up at me. "And I'm going home to him tonight."

So we had dinner but finally, after we'd finished eating, I got up my nerve and asked the question. "What about your fantasy?"

Nancy looked at me for a while. "Maybe Charlie has a hidden fantasy like I did," she said at last. "If he does, then I can spend the rest of my life exploring it with him, just like you did with me." Then she smiled at me.

"I hope I'm as good at it as you were," she said.

7

Bonny
("Psychological Masochist")

I met Bonny the first week after she moved to New York from Philadelphia to begin her new job as a media buyer at the advertising agency I was then working for. Bonny was twenty-seven years old and very
pretty, with long dark blonde hair cut in a pageboy, blue eyes, and
a body that finally, much to Bonny's displeasure, I labeled as
"sturdy" . . . not at all fat but not thin, either. Just big-boned and solid
with strong shoulders, beautiful breasts, and a sensational ass.

Of course, I didn't know any of this when I first saw Bonny walking down the hall outside my office. She was simply new and attractive and pleasant and friendly, so I introduced myself, invited her to
lunch the next day, and then to dinner two nights later.

I rarely make love to a "straight" girl on a first date. In S/M activities I am totally dominant and sexually self-assured, and sex in virtu-
ally any form is a natural and even automatic part of any relationship
with a submissive. But outside of the "scene," I tend to move quite
slowly with women—almost shyly; my approach to sex is usually quite
careful and even awkward at times. (It has occurred to me more than
once that this difference is a very major factor in the appeal that S/M
holds for me.)

But Bonny made it very easy. After dinner we went back to her apartment. She turned on the stereo, poured us both brandy, kicked off her shoes, and curled up next to me on the couch, leaning her head on my shoulder. When I kissed her she opened her mouth, teased my tongue with hers, and turned to wrap one arm tightly around my neck. When I put one hand on her waist, she covered it with her own hand and firmly moved it to her breast, holding it there. After a while Bonny got up to pour two more brandies. Before returning to the couch she casually stripped off her blouse and skirt, and a while later, when I suggested that we might move to her bedroom, she said simply, "Of course."

It was very good and very easy and very natural. We took time to undress each other slowly, and then spent a long time touching and kissing each other, sort of exploring each other's bodies. I went down on her and used my tongue to bring her to orgasm. Then she said, "My turn," rolled me onto my back, and began expertly licking and sucking my cock. But before I came I stopped her, rolled her over, and put my cock into her very ready pussy, and we made love that way slowly and gently for a long time. She came again before I did, and afterward we dozed for a while with our arms around each other.

I woke up when Bonny got up to go to the bathroom. When she came back, I asked her to bring me another brandy. She did, and then sat next to me on the bed, touching me lightly now and then while we talked about our jobs and when we were kids and all sorts of things.

I never did find out exactly what made Bonny decide to do what she did next; but after we had talked for more than an hour, she said she wanted to show me something. She got up, went over to the dresser, knelt down, and pulled open the bottom drawer. She rummaged through it for a minute, then stood up and turned around. She was holding a whip.

It was exactly like the braided cat-o'-nine-tails that I had bought to use on Paula, except it was light brown instead of black. Bonny was holding the handle in her right hand and the nine lashes in her left, sort of stretching the whip out. She walked over and stood next to the bed.

Sometimes I'm not too clever at conversation. "It's a whip," I said at last.

"That's right."

"I've got one like it," I told her.

"I thought you might have," Bonny said. I didn't answer. "Would you do me a favor and use it on me?" she asked."

"Of course," I agreed.

Bonny lay on the bed, face down, pulled a pillow under her head, and spread her arms and legs. She took a grip on the end of the mattress and turned her head to look at me. "Please whip my ass," she said. "You don't have to be gentle. I can take quite a lot."

I began, whipping her slowly and steadily, delivering a stroke about every five seconds or so. After maybe twenty lashes, Bonny buried her face in the pillow and tightened her grip on the bed. She began moving her body, slowly grinding her hips and clenching her fingers each time the whip came down on her ass. After about forty lashes, she began to jump each time the whip fell and I heard her making a soft crying sound which wasn't quite muffled by the pillow. I asked her if she wanted me to stop but she shook her head without looking up.

I lost count of the times I swung the whip across her naked bottom, which by now was a solid bright pink with many dark red and purple welts that I knew would last for several days. Finally Bonny lifted her head from the pillow and turned to look at me. Her face was covered with tears.

"I'm sorry," I heard her say. "I'm sorry . . . I'm sorry. Please don't punish me any more."

I stopped immediately.

I dropped the whip on the floor and sat on the bed next to her. I stroked Bonny's head and her back, and when she turned onto her side I kissed her. I got a washcloth and bathed her face; she kissed my hand and smiled at me.

"Thank you," she said.

"Want to tell me what that was all about?" I asked.

"Not now," Bonny said. "But it would be really nice if you'd stay here and let me suck you off and then hold me and let me go to sleep that way."

I could hardly refuse.

Bonny was already up when I awoke the next morning. I called to her and she came into the bedroom wearing a bathrobe and carrying a cup of coffee.

"Are you OK?" I asked.

She smiled and bent over and kissed me lightly. "Sure," she said. "Let me see your bottom."

Bonny put the coffee cup down on the dresser, turned around, and pulled the robe up to her waist. Her ass was covered with purple and red bruises. It looked awful.

"Holy shit!" I said.

Bonny dropped the robe and turned around. the smiled again and nodded her head. "Yeah," she agreed, "that was a pretty good job you did. I'm going to have a little trouble sitting down today."

"I'm sorry," I told her.

Bonny knelt next to the bed, leaned over to put her hand on my cheek, and kissed me again. She looked very serious. "Please don't be sorry," she said. "I really need that once in a while. You did me a favor. Honest." She paused and went on: "Of course, I took a little more last night than usual."

"How come?" I asked.

Bonny grinned at me. "I sort of had the feeling you were enjoying it, too," she said.

I had to go on a business trip the next day, so I didn't see Bonny the rest of the week or over the weekend. But on Monday I went by her office and we made a date for dinner the next night. We went to a Chinese place down on Mott Street and then home to her apartment where we made love most of the night. But nothing else happened and I didn't talk about the whipping. Two nights later we went to a movie and again spent the night together without any talk about what had happened.

But on Wednesday of the following week, I was sitting in my office when suddenly I looked up and saw Bonny standing in the doorway. "You busy tomorrow night?" she asked.

"No."

"Could I cook you dinner?"

"Sure."

"Good," Bonny said. Then she studied her toes for a few seconds before looking up at me again. She seemed embarrassed. Finally she spoke. "After dinner I think I'm going to need some help again," she said, and before I could answer she turned and quickly walked away.

Since I'd gotten hung up in a late meeting Thursday, Bonny went on home without me and I got there about an hour later. Bonny came to the door in bare feet, her hair tied back in a ponytail, wearing blue jeans and nothing else. God, she was beautiful!

She was cooking an Italian veal dish, and handed me a glass of red wine as I sat on the couch and watched her move back and forth from the kitchen to the dining area. I think it was the first time I ever got turned on by a woman's back, but hers was absolutely beautiful, with strong wide shoulders tapering to a tight waist. I couldn't help thinking about the kind of whipping a big strong girl like her might be able to take. I think that's when I first called her "sturdy." She swatted me on the head and huffed for a while, but later she kissed me.

Bonny stayed dressed that way during dinner. I sat across from her trying to concentrate on the food, but her breasts kept demanding my attention. They were "strong," too, very rounded and full, about a B, I guessed, with almost no sag at all. Bonny continued to act totally calm while I was having all sorts of trouble. Finally I couldn't take it any more.

"Jesus Christ!" I said. "You are absolutely driving me stark raving fucking nuts!"

Bonny looked up and grinned. "I thought you'd never notice," she said.

"It's unfair," I grumbled.

Bonny laughed. "Of course it's unfair, but I plan to take advantage of you later, so I need you off guard."

"I'm ready to be taken advantage of right now," I told her.

"Patience, John, patience," Bonny answered. I went back to trying to play it cool but it sure as hell wasn't easy.

After dinner I moved back to the couch while Bonny made espresso. Later she sat on the floor next to my feet and put her head in my lap and her arms around my waist while I gently stroked her back. After a while, without raising her head, Bonny started talking.

"Do you remember the first night you were here?"

"Sure."

"Did you have a good time?"

"I loved making love to you," I answered.

"I mean while you were whipping me."

"Yes," I admitted.

Bonny looked up at me for a minute, then put her head back in my lap and gave me a quick hug. "You've whipped other girls, haven't you?" But she already knew the answer to that question.

"Yes, I have."

"Good," Bonny said. "Some day I'm going to get you to tell me all about them, but now I need your help."

"What kind of help?" I asked.

"Don't act dumb," Bonny said. She stood up, took my hand, pulled me to my feet, and led me into the bedroom. There she turned around and unbuttoned my shirt, pulling it wide open, and then she put her arms around my neck and pressed her body against mine so that those marvelous breasts flattened against my chest. She kissed me long and hard, and then tucked her face into my shoulder and began talking.

"Will you do it my way?" she whispered.

Hugging her, I said I would.

Bonny stripped off her jeans and panties, went to the dresser, and got the whip. Then she went to the closet, and when she turned around she was holding four very long and heavy inch-wide woven luggage straps. Finally she opened a drawer in the little bedside table and took out a ball gag—a small red rubber ball with a heavy leather thong running through the middle of it. I'd never seen one before except in a picture, but I knew what it was.

I guess I looked a little strange because Bonny came back and hugged me again. "Don't worry," she told me. "I know what I'm doing."

Bonny let me go and sat on the edge of the bed, tying a strap around each of her ankles with the buckle close to the knot so that most of the strap was left free. Then she asked me to tie the other two straps to her wrists in the same way. She explained that I should pass each strap around a leg of the bed and bring it back up and through the buckle. That way, by simply pulling on the end of each strap, I could stretch her as tightly as I wanted.

When we were ready, she lay on her belly, tucked a pillow under her head, spread her legs, and held out her arms. "Tie me really tight," she told me. I did.

When I was finished tying her, Bonny asked me to sit on the bed next to her and she turned her head so that she could look at me. "I want you to remember that you promised to do what I asked," she said.

"I remember."

Bonny nodded. "Good," she said. "Do you remember how many times you whipped me last time?"

I shook my head.

"Eighty-seven," Bonny told me. "Now, what I want is for you to use that gag and tie it really tight. And then I want you to whip me one hundred and fifty times."

"For Christ's sake!" I said. "*Last* time was too much."

Bonny shook her head. "No it wasn't, and tonight I need more. That's why I picked a Thursday. I'm going to call in sick tomorrow; that way I'll have three days to rest."

I started to argue but Bonny wouldn't let me. "You promised, didn't you?"

"Maybe I shouldn't have," I told her.

"But you did and you'll keep it, right?"

I stared at her for a while. "OK," I said finally.

"Good," Bonny said. "And just one more very important thing. Even with the gag and the pillow I'll probably make a lot of noise." She stopped and took a deep breath. "But I want you to promise that no matter what I do, you won't stop and you won't start taking it easy. I want you to whip me as hard as you did last time, and no matter if I scream or cry or even faint, don't stop before one hundred and fifty."

"Are you absolutely sure?" I asked her one more time.

"Absolutely," she answered.

First I kissed her. Next I put the gag in her mouth, tying it as tightly as I could. Then I pulled each of the four straps even tighter, so that her body was stretched to its limits.

I began the whipping. I used the same tempo as I had that first night, bringing the nine heavy braided lashes down across her ass in a slow, deliberate, steady rhythm. For the first fifteen or twenty lashes Bonny remained completely motionless. During the next twenty or so her hips began to move in that grinding motion I'd seen the first night, except that, tied as she was, she couldn't move as much.

I had counted the fiftieth stroke before I heard Bonny make the first noise; but after that, each time the whip fell, I heard a little scream through the gag while her fingers would clench into a fist, then open again. Even tied the way she was, Bonny's entire body would jump with the pain.

I kept going, bringing the braided leather strands down hard at the same pace so that she could anticipate each stroke and I could see her body tighten just a split second before each one. By the time I was halfway through, Bonny was screaming steadily through the gag, twisting her head back and forth violently and fighting with all her strength against the straps that held her to the bed.

By the time I reached a hundred lashes, her ass looked awful— even worse than it had that first night. Bonny was making a terrible noise and now she was literally whipping her head back and forth each time the whip landed. She was crying and tears were running down her cheeks, soaking the pillow.

"Do you want me to stop?" I asked, pausing for a minute.

Bonny nodded her head "yes" emphatically, and I heard her desperately trying to say "please" through the gag.

After looking at her for several minutes, I finally made up my mind. "A promise is a promise," I said.

I took the three cushions and two large throw pillows from the living room couch and brought them back to the bedroom. Piling them over her head, I then took a heavy blanket, folded it, and draped it over the pillows to hold them in place. Even so, as I started the whipping again, Bonny's screams came through clearly.

I whipped her ass ten more times, but then I decided that I hadn't promised to whip only her ass, so I began whipping her back instead. After fifteen lashes that beautiful strong back was covered with welts from her shoulders to her waist, but I kept going for a total of thirty.

"Ten more," I said at last, and for those final ten strokes I moved back to her ass, swinging the heavy whip as hard as I could, almost driving her body into the bed. With three lashes left to go, Bonny suddenly stopped screaming and her body relaxed, but I finished anyway, counting out loud, "one-forty-eight, one-forty-nine, one-fifty!"

When I pulled the blanket and pillows away, I found that Bonny had fainted.

I removed the gag from her mouth and loosened the straps on her wrists and ankles, leaving them still tied but giving her some slack so that she could move if she wanted to. I got a damp towel and bathed her face, and then I just sat next to her.

After two or three minutes Bonny moved. She buried her head in the pillow and let out a little moan; she moved her arms until she felt the straps still tied to them. She began to cry again and through the crying I heard her say, "Oh please, Daddy, oh please! I'm sorry, Daddy! Please don't punish me any more, please! I won't do it again, Daddy. I promise. Please don't whip me any more!"

I took hold of her hair and gently turned her head. Her eyes were shut tight and she was sobbing. I kissed her, then kissed her again. She opened her eyes and looked at me, sort of blankly at first and then, with a sudden start, her eyes focused.

"It's me," I said. "It's me, Bonny. I'm John. It's me."

She began crying again, but this time it sounded more like a cry of relief. After a while she stopped crying and I washed her face again.

"Is it over?" Bonny asked after a few minutes.

"Yes."

"Did you really whip me one hundred and fifty times?"

I nodded my head. "Every one," I told her.

"You knew I wanted you to stop, didn't you?" she asked me.

"Yes, I did."

"But you didn't," she said.

"I promised you I wouldn't."

Bonny lay there looking at me. "That's why I picked you," she said at last. "I knew you'd have enough guts to go all the way."

After I'd untied her, Bonny took a shower. Since she was pretty shaky, I helped her, gently washing her back and her ass, being as careful as I could. But it still hurt like hell, especially when the soap burned the places where her skin had been broken.

Afterward, she lay on the bed while I rubbed vitamin E cream all over her back and rear end, which was really a mess. Bonny told me that the cream would help her heal more quickly, but I knew that no matter what she did she'd have the marks for days.

Finally, Bonny curled up in my arms and we fell asleep that way without making love. However, the next morning I woke up with the lovely feeling of Bonny's mouth and tongue slowly moving on my cock. I put my hand on her head to let her know I was awake. She reached up and squeezed it, then kept on slowly and carefully and very expertly sucking my cock until I climaxed.

She kept her mouth on me for a while after I came, and then she moved up on the bed and kissed me. "That's my way of saying thank you," she said. "I wanted to do it last night after you untied me but I was too tired."

"I love your doing that," I told her, "but you don't have to thank me for anything."

"I owe you a lot more than you know," she said.

We left it there. I helped Bonny cook breakfast and afterward I put more of the cream on her back. It looked even worse than the night before, covered with large ugly black, blue, and purple bruises in addition to the many vivid red marks where the whip had cut the skin a little.

"I hope you don't do this very often," I told her.

"Not like that, I don't," she said. But she was smiling.

"I think it's about time you told me about it," I said to her.

"Me, too," Bonny agreed. "Let's go for a walk."

We walked over to the park next to the United Nations Building and sat on a bench looking at the East River. After a long time, Bonny told me the story. It was really pretty simple.

It seems that Bonny had a brother. He was seven years older than she was and she had worshiped him from the day she was born. One day, when she was six and her brother thirteen, they started fooling around. One thing led to another, and finally Bonny wound up on her knees sucking on her brother's penis. Neither of them had any real idea of what they were doing.

Their mother caught them, of course, and was hysterical; and when her mother told her father, he reacted the same way, only more violently. He took them both down to the cellar, tied them to two separate support posts, and whipped them both with a belt. While he beat them, he kept telling them how sick and filthy and horrible they were, and that God would also punish them, and that neither he nor their mother nor God would ever forgive them.

All during the remainder of her childhood and adolescence, Bonny's father kept at it. He constantly reminded her of how "evil" she was and used his belt on her at the slightest provocation. He never stopped until he died of a heart attack when Bonny was sixteen; but even then it wasn't over because her mother kept it going. Although her mother didn't beat her, she did take every opportunity to tell Bonny that she had caused her father's heart attack by being such an evil person.

Bonny turned to look at me. "It was awful but it was weird, too," she said. "It didn't mess me up in other ways like you'd think it would have. I learned that I loved sex with the right kind of men, and I did OK at school and everything. But I never got over it."

"I went to college," she told me. "I was eighteen then. The first month there I met a boy who reminded me of my brother and I slept with him on our second date. He was the first one and I loved doing it and I thought I loved him. But after three weeks, I felt this terrible guilt and finally one night I asked him to spank me. That's the last I ever saw of him."

"I went to the college shrink for a while," Bonny continued, "and then I went to another one a couple of years ago in Philadelphia, but neither of them ever did me much good." She turned and stared out at the river. "Hell, I knew why I was the way I was, so what could they tell me?" She shrugged her shoulders. "I guess that after being told you're evil and deserve to be punished for almost twelve years, you just sort of believe it."

"But you know it's not true," I argued. "Shit, you were only six years old!"

"I know," Bonny said, "but it still doesn't help. It just builds up in me and builds and builds, and finally I just have to have someone do that to me."

"Whip you?" I asked.

"Punish me," Bonny said.

We sat there for a while with our arms around each other, watching the boats on the river. Finally Bonny reached out and took my hand, squeezing it while I looked at her. She reached over with her other hand, holding mine in both of hers, and smiled at me. "At least there's one thing good," she said.

"What's that?"

"I've found out that the longer and harder I'm punished, the longer I can go before I need it again. That's why I asked you to do that last night."

"It's just as well," I told her. "I don't think either of us could handle that too often." I squeezed her hand back. "How long do you figure last night will keep you?"

"I don't know," Bonny said. "That's the most I've ever had. The most before that was a couple of years ago in Philadelphia and after that I didn't do anything for about six weeks."

"How many lashes was it that time?" I asked.

"A hundred," she said, "but not as hard as you did last night. You're the first man I've ever met who I thought was strong enough and, well, dominant enough to really give me a chance to take me as far as I need to go."

"So this one ought to last a couple of months," I suggested.

"We'll see," Bonny said.

It lasted three weeks.

I had asked Bonny to go to dinner and she showed up late. She also acted fairly shitty during dinner, and later at her apartment she did or said something that really pissed me off. I don't remember what it was but I was really mad, and finally I yanked her down across my lap and spanked her as hard as I could. She fought and yelled and cried, but I didn't stop until she said she was sorry for the way she'd behaved.

Afterward we went to bed and made love. It wasn't until later, while I was holding her and drifting off to sleep, that I suddenly realized that Bonny had conned me into the spanking.

"You're a bitch!" I told her, but she knew I wasn't mad.

"You're a pushover," Bonny giggled, and then she pushed me onto my back and took my cock into her warm and expert mouth. She was right. I was a pushover.

Bonny and I dated for about eight months and after a while it seemed that we only went out when Bonny felt the need to be "punished." I told her about some of the things I'd done with other "slaves" and once in a while we would try something different. One time I took her out in the country, tied her to a tree, and whipped her; another time I tied her with her hands over her head, and slowly and methodically tormented her breasts, using a whip and clothespins. Bonny took this for quite a while, but finally she begged me to stop. Then she asked me to tie her to the bed and whip her ass the way I usually did.

And invariably, whenever I "punished" her, Bonny would finally come to a point where she would "break." I'd hear her crying and whispering, "Please don't punish me any more. Please. I'm sorry. I won't do it again. Please don't punish me any more."

And afterward she would almost always use her mouth on me until I climaxed.

It ended abruptly. It was a night when Bonny wanted to be really punished to her limits. I had tied and gagged her and, working more slowly than usual, had whipped her ass and her back and her legs a total of two hundred times—the number she had set. Bonny screamed into the gag and pillows all through the last hundred lashes; when I finally finished and removed the gag, I heard her start the now familiar litany:

"I'm sorry . . . I'm sorry. Please don't whip me any more. Please. Robby, please. I won't do it again. I'm sorry, Robby. Please don't punish me any more."

After she calmed down I untied her. She knelt between my legs and began her ritual of blowing me. Suddenly I stopped her. "Who's Robby?" I asked her.

Bonny looked up at me, startled. "I don't understand," she said.

"Robby," I repeated. "When I took the gag out you said, 'I'm sorry, Robby.' "

Bonny knelt up straight and stared at me. She had absolutely no expression whatsoever on her face. "Robby's my brother," she said at last.

"Oh," I said. "I don't think you ever told me his name."

As a matter of fact, I realized then that she had never mentioned him at all except that one time in the park when she had told me the story about what had happened. "Where's Robby now?" I asked.

Bonny's face went white. Her body was rigid, and she started to tremble, and then she began to cry harder than I had ever seen her cry before, almost hysterically. She curled her fingers into fists and pressed them hard against her temples for a minute. Suddenly she began using them to pound me on the chest and face and belly while she kept screaming, "No, you son of a bitch! No! No! No! No, you goddamn dirty son of a bitch!"

I grabbed her before she could hurt me, rolled her over, and pinned her to the bed. "What the hell is the matter?" I yelled at her.

Bonny's face was filled with fury. "You dirty fucking son of a bitch!" she snarled. "You fucking bastard! You had to ask about him, didn't you?"

"You mean Robby?" I asked.

Bonny was fighting to get loose. "Yes, you son of a bitch!"

"What about Robby?" I asked.

Bonny stopped struggling and looked up at me. Her teeth were clenched and there was nothing but pure hate in her eyes. Finally she spoke.

"Robby hung himself in the garage two days after it happened," she said. "Now get the fuck out of here!"

I didn't know what to say or do. I let go of Bonny, who curled up into a ball and began crying softly. I dressed as quickly as I could and left. But before I was gone, I heard her begin talking again and I will never forget, as long as I live, the pain and desperation in Bonny's voice as she whispered over and over again, "I'm sorry, Robby. I'm sorry . . . I'm sorry . . . I'm sorry."

8

Vanessa
("The Challenger")

Excerpt from a letter from Vanessa

I have a fantasy. You have taken me to the basement of a large house somewhere, and you have tied me naked and spread-eagled . . . my arms stretched high over my head with my wrists bound with leather straps to rings bolted to the huge rough wooden beams of the ceiling . . . my legs spread wide and ankles chained to rings set in the stone floor. I know you are planning to "test" me again with your hands and your whips but tonight I feel very strong.

So as soon as you finish with the chains I tell you that before you begin my torment I have something that I want to say to you. These are my words:

"John, I feel very sturdy and very brave tonight and I think it is time for me to try something that I've thought about for a long time . . . the 'ultimate' game.

"The way I feel I don't think you're tough enough or cruel enough to 'break' me no matter what you do. But I'm going to give you three hours to prove I'm wrong, and if I don't 'break' then I win a prize.

"The prize is you . . . in a soundproof room, tied in any way I choose,

with every *kind of whip and torture device I can think of,* and no time limit at all! *And I get to see how long it takes to break* you."

And then I laugh and throw my head back, arching my breasts toward your whip, and I wait for my test of torture to begin.

Needless to say, I never gave Vanessa the chance. But on occasions I did "break" her. It was never easy.

Vanessa is a petite, slender, and pretty woman. She is only five feet two inches tall, with lovely long red hair and a thin body that she keeps in excellent shape. When we met, Vanessa was twenty-seven years old and worked in the personnel department of an airline. She was single and lived alone in an apartment on Central Park West.

I met Vanessa one bitter-cold January night at the "Cattleman" restaurant across the street from the building where I was working then.

We both arrived at the front door at the same time. I opened it for her, commented on the lousy weather, and received a smile and a pleasant answer in return. As soon as we got inside the lobby, I asked her if she was meeting someone. She said no, neither was I, and I suggested that we go to the bar together. In response I got a long, obviously appraising look and finally a nod.

"You just might be good enough," she said. "Let's find out." She turned around so I could take her coat, and when I came back from the check room she reached out to shake my hand. "My name's Vanessa M_____," she told me, "and I'm frequently a pain in the ass, so if I start getting bitchy don't take it personally." With that she took my arm and we went on into the bar. I hadn't even told her my name yet.

But five hours later, when I put Vanessa in a cab and headed on home alone, we each had a pretty good idea of who the other one was, and just where we might be heading together.

That first night we started with several drinks at the bar, crowded as always with singles looking for companionship. She told me about her job and I told her about mine. We talked about sports—she swam and rode horses, I played golf and tennis. And then we talked about books, movies, politics, music, and just about everything else.

Vanessa was "pushing" all the way. Was I good at my job? How well did I play golf? Had I read the latest book? What about the latest "hot" movie? Did I know who Billie Holiday was? It wasn't unpleasant. It wasn't exactly fun, either. But it sure as hell kept me awake.

Eventually we got a table for dinner and I began to push back.

Why was she still in a clerical position if she had a college degree? If she knew so much about Dixieland jazz how come she'd never heard of George Brunis? Were those shoes of hers really still in style? Why didn't she have a date?

It didn't register with her at first; but after a while, right in the middle of answering one of my questions, she suddenly stopped talking and looked at me hard. At first I thought she was angry, but then she grinned and shook her head slowly. "You sneaky son of a bitch!" she said. "You really had me going! That's pretty damn good. I think you may be a 'keeper.' "

After that, the pressure was off. We both relaxed and enjoyed our dinner and some good conversation. We went back to the bar for a couple of drinks after dinner and finally, at about ten o'clock, it was time to leave. I had already established the fact that I was married and had to get home, but I did offer to see her safely into a cab.

I flagged down a passing taxi and held the door for her. She gave me a quick but very thorough kiss, at the same time pressing her breast against my arm, and then she got into the back seat. Just before I closed the door, Vanessa looked up and winked at me. "I'd like a rematch," she said.

"You got it," I answered.

We went out again two or three weeks later, and again we both went home alone. But it was a fine evening with a lot of verbal sparring—a sort of long, gentle "try to get one up" session. A lot of fun, a lot of laughs, and another very sexy goodnight kiss.

I took her home on our third date, and we spent a lot of time touching and kissing; but even that was sort of a challenge—a contest to see who would suggest going to bed first. Neither of us did. But when I finally left at close to one in the morning, Vanessa was obviously ready and willing, and when I kissed her good night she ground her pelvis against my erection. Then she stepped back, gave me that same grin, and reached out to shake my hand.

"You're pretty tough," she said. "Don't change."

I shook her hand and left without comment.

On the next date we had hamburgers at Allen's and went to an early movie. All through the film Vanessa had her hand on mine or else on my arm or thigh, and finally, near the end of the movie, she very firmly put her hand on my crotch and began stroking my cock through the cloth of my slacks. Somehow I managed to not show any response. I didn't squirm. I didn't even breathe hard. She kept it up during the cab ride back to her apartment and still I acted as if nothing were happening. Of course, I couldn't very well hide the fact that I was hard as a rock.

But as soon as the apartment door closed behind us, I slammed Vanessa up against the wall, pinning both her wrists behind her with one hand while my other hand wrapped itself in that long red hair, yanking her head back and holding it motionless. I kissed her as hard and as brutally as I could, deliberately trying to hurt her. I ground my mouth down so that my teeth were bruising her lips painfully as well as mine, and I slowly tightened the grip on her hair until I knew it must be hurting her.

I finally let go of her wrists, but I kept her pinned against the wall with one hip so that her arms were still held behind her. I unbuttoned her coat, jacket, and blouse and I pulled her bra up to expose her breasts. I ran my hand over both of them roughly, squeezing and kneading them and pinching the hard nipples. Vanessa kept her eyes closed and never flinched.

Still holding her by the hair, I slipped her skirt and panties down in one motion so that they were around her knees, and I rammed a finger into her pussy. She was very wet and when I pressed even harder into her, I felt her pushing back with her hips.

Neither of us had said a word. I kissed her again, this time using my free hand to force her mouth open. When I felt her tongue flick into my mouth, I caught it with my teeth and bit it until I felt her whole body react to the pain.

Pulling down on her hair to force her to her knees, I unzipped my fly and took out my hardened cock. Vanessa finally took her hands from behind her back and used them to cup my testicles and hold the base of my erection while I forced it deep into her mouth.

Her tongue and lips worked together, and very quickly I was ready to come. Vanessa must have felt the tension building in me because suddenly, despite the painful grip I had on her hair, she twisted her head to one side, away from my cock.

"Please," she said. "You can come in my mouth any time you want, but the first time I want you inside me. Please!"

I hauled Vanessa to her feet and, still using her hair to hold her, I half dragged her into the living room. Along the way she managed to kick off her skirt, panties, and shoes and to drop the coat and jacket from her shoulders. But she was still wearing her blouse and her bra. Leading her to a large stuffed armchair, I roughly forced her to bend forward over the back of it. I let go of her hair at last and quickly removed my slacks and shorts. I then took one of her wrists in each hand, holding them tightly behind her and using her arms as levers to keep her bent over the chair. She spread her legs without my having to ask her.

"Say 'please' again," I ordered her.

"Please," she whispered.

I went into her hard from behind, but I pumped my cock very slowly, trying to last as long as I could. Vanessa couldn't move too much the way I was holding her, but she did as much as she could, grinding her hips and ass to heighten her own pleasure as well as mine. Finally I heard saying, "Oh, yes, yes, yes, yes, yes! yes! yes! YES! YES! YES! YES!"

That did it for me. I pulled my cock almost free of her cunt and then rammed it back into her as hard as I possibly could, maybe ten times while she continued to scream, "YES! YES! YES! YES!" and then I came, too.

I woke up in the middle of the night to feel Vanessa's mouth on my nipple. I lay still while she slowly worked her way down across my belly to my cock. I continued to lie there, unmoving, while she began gently sucking me and I let her keep at it until I was almost ready to come. Then I put my hand gently on the back of her head and stroked her a couple of times before I grabbed her hair in my fist and used it to hold her head motionless while I exploded deep into her throat.

"That was lovely," I said afterwards.

"You deserved it," Vanessa said. "You're the first man who's made me say 'please' in years."

It was two or three dates later that the subject of S/M first came up. We were quietly talking and undressing for bed at Vanessa's apartment, and I had pulled my belt out and wrapped one end around my right fist.

"You hold that belt like a whip," Vanessa commented.

"I've used it as a whip now and then," I answered.

"You've whipped people?" she asked. I nodded. "Women?"

"*Only* women," I told her.

When Vanessa had finished undressing, she put on her bathrobe and curled up on her side of the bed, patting the space next to her in a gesture that invited me to sit beside her. "Tell me about it," she asked.

I told her about Carol in Chicago and Nancy and Bonny, and some of the other submissive women I'd been with. I didn't give her all the details. Deliberately leaving out the rougher parts, I tried to concentrate on the sensuality and excitement. Vanessa asked several questions along the way, mainly probing for details about how the various women had reacted to what I had done to them. Had they screamed? Did they cry? Did they get turned on? Did they ever faint? Did any of them ever beg me to stop?

Finally there wasn't much left for me to tell, and Vanessa began talking. "I don't think being whipped would turn me on," she said. "I think I'd love doing that to a man, though, particularly some really big guy like a football player, maybe. God, I'd like to work over some huge jock type and watch him cry and beg! What a kick that would be!" She paused and looked at me thoughtfully for a while. "Of course, even though I don't think I'd turn on to pain, it's sort of exciting to think about, and God knows I was more turned on that night you more or less raped me in the living room than I have ever been in my life! But I don't think it was the pain, it was just having a really strong man forcing me to do whatever he wanted, and you didn't really hurt me that much. It was just pure animal sex!" She leaned over and kissed me. "I really loved it!"

"But I don't think pain would be very sexy," she continued. Then she paused and looked at me. "But the idea of proving to myself that I could take it, *that* could be exciting." Then she grinned at me. "And maybe proving it to someone else, too."

"Did you have anyone in mind?" I asked.

Vanessa stuck her tongue out at me. "Yeah," she said, "Kirk Douglas, but you'll have to do."

"You want me to whip you?" I asked.

"That's not the way I want to think about it," Vanessa said. "It's more just in my head. I mean it's not so much that I want you to whip me. Instead it's that I'd like to see if I could take it." She sort of smiled to herself. "Does that make any sense?" she asked.

"I'm not sure," I told her, "but I guess I understand."

"Then will you do it?" she asked. "I mean right now would you tie me up and whip me with that belt?

I thought for a while. "I'll tell you what," I said finally. "I'll do it, but I'll do it my way. You take off that robe and lie on your tummy. You spread your arms and legs out and hold onto the head of the bed and don't move. But I won't tie you. Not this time, at least."

Vanessa did what I had told her to do and then turned her head to look at me. "Now," I said, "I'm going to use the belt on you. I don't know how hard or how long . . . just whatever I feel like."

"Why won't you tie me?" Vanessa asked.

"Because that way you can stop it if you want to," I explained. "If you find out that you've made a mistake, or if it gets too much for you, you can just get up." Then I grinned at her. "Of course, there's another way you can stop it," I said.

"How's that?" she asked.

"Just say, 'please,' " I told her.

Vanessa looked at me for a long time. "You play dirty," she said at last. Then she buried her head in the pillow. "Any time," I heard her mumble. After moving her long, lovely red hair so that it wouldn't cover her back, I began.

I had deliberately decided not to make her say "please." Instead I whipped her very carefully and very slowly, giving her plenty of time between the lashes to get ready for the next one, and moving the belt each time so that I never hit her twice in a row in the same place. Ass, back, legs, shoulders, thighs, and then around again, but in a different pattern. I also changed the intensity—two or three moderate lashes, then a couple of very light ones, and then maybe a very hard one. But here, too, I changed the pattern so that Vanessa never knew where the next stroke of my belt would land or how hard it would be.

Vanessa lay almost still most of the time. On a few of the harder lashes she would jump slightly and sort of hunch her shoulders if the belt had struck her back, or else clench the muscles of her ass if that part of her body had been the target. But she never made a sound.

After maybe forty or fifty lashes I stopped, but I did make the last three or four quite hard, and on the last one Vanessa jerked her head back in reaction to the pain. I gently dragged the belt up and down over her back a couple of times, slowly caressing her body with the leather from her shoulders to her ankles. Then I lay the belt down across her back.

"That's it," I told her

Vanessa lay quietly for a while, then rolled over and sat up on the bed. She picked up the belt, fingered it, and then looked at me. "How did I do?" she asked.

"You tell me," I answered.

Vanessa got up and crossed the room to the dresser, twisting her head to examine her back in the mirror, studying the wide red marks that covered most of her body. Finally she turned back to me.

"I think I did pretty good," she told me, and then she smiled. "And you didn't make me say 'please,' " she added. She lay down on the bed again, this time on her back, and she spread her legs and reached up with her arms, signaling for me to join her. "Hurry up," she said. "I feel very proud and very sexy."

I stripped quickly and started into bed, but Vanessa held up her hand. "One more thing," she said. "Since I won the game, you have to eat me first."

I didn't argue, and as excited as she was it didn't take long to make her scream . . . not from pain but from pure animal pleasure.

We went on from there. It didn't happen on every date as it would have with a true submissive. Instead, on maybe every third or fourth date, Vanessa would say something like, "I feel pretty tough tonight," or I would say, "I think I'm in a mood to see if I can make you beg." And if it turned out that we were both in the mood, as usually it would, we'd have a session.

Most of the time I'd stop on purpose before Vanessa gave in. But once in a while I'd deliberately "break" her, just to make sure that she understood that I could any time I really wanted to. But even then it was never easy, and with Vanessa continuously raising the ante, these games of ours produced some pretty memorable times.

Excerpt from a note from Vanessa

My latest fantasy concerns my birthday present to you. In this fantasy I have asked you to tie me by my thumbs and to pull me up until only the tips of my toes are touching the floor and most of my weight is on my thumbs. My ankles are strapped together to make it harder for me to balance. I have asked you to take that special whip that produces only light marks but such great *pain, and I have asked you to whip only* my breasts and belly, *because I know that whipping those parts of my body gives you the most pleasure.*

Finally, I have told you that I want very much for you to whip me for as long as I can possibly stand it, and that I will count for you and that each time I say another number you are to whip me again.

I know how much pleasure each one will give you, and I have determined to count for as long as I possibly can.

I hear my voice . . . "nine hundred and fifty-nine," and I wonder if your arm is getting tired.

Another time, much more recently, Vanessa and I wound up at my SoHo apartment with two other dominant men. Earlier in the evening there had also been two other submissive women and a male slave present, and all of us, including Vanessa, had spent several hours engaged in a carefully planned and quite heavy program of submission and discipline.

But now the two other "slaves" were gone, leaving Vanessa and me alone with the two men. I allowed one of the other men to take her from behind while she performed expert fellatio on me—an arrangement we both occasionally enjoyed—but he had climaxed and had gone into the bathroom, leaving Vanessa to continue pleasing me.

As soon as we were alone, Vanessa removed her mouth from my cock and looked at me with an expression that I knew, from much experience, meant that she was feeling adventurous. "Are you in a hurry?" she asked me.

"Not particularly."

"Good," Vanessa said. "Those guys thought their two 'slaves' were pretty tough. I'd like to show them what a *real* woman can take. Besides, since I was mostly in a dominant role tonight, physically at least, it ought to blow their minds to see you discipline me. But I mean *for real!*"

"Just how high up for it are you?" I asked her.

"High as a kite, lover," Vanessa told me. "I'm ready for a truly heavy show."

"Name it," I told her.

"Good. First, I want you to hang me up by the wrists. Then I want you to put two needles into each of my breasts—one on each side. And then I want you to whip me, just as hard as you can, fifty times. And finally, when you're finished, I want you to leave me hanging there and show our guests out. And I want you to explain to them that now you're going to start getting *really* heavy and that the things you have planned would best be done in private. Their imaginations ought to do the rest." She paused and grinned at me. "And if you do that," she added, "I'll suck your cock the whole rest of the night."

"What the hell got into you?" I asked her.

Vanessa flashed me one of her patented grins. "I popped two amyl nitrates while you weren't looking," she confessed. "I won't even feel it."

She was wrong, of course.

First, I put *four* needles into each of her breasts. Then I whipped her a *hundred* times before asking the other two men to leave. And finally, when we were alone, instead of untying her, I left her hanging there while I poured myself a brandy and then made myself comfortable on the couch.

Vanessa's head was thrown back and her eyes were closed. Most of her body, with the exception of her breasts, was covered with the marks of the whipping I'd given her. But she had never made a sound the entire time.

After a minute or two she picked up her head and opened her eyes, and when she saw me sitting there on the couch, holding a brandy, it registered on her. But she never lost control.

"Not bad," she muttered. "I did a number on them and now you're doing a number on me."

"That's right," I agreed, raising the brandy snifter in salute.

"When does it end?" she asked.

"Whenever you say 'please,' " I told her.

Vanessa looked at me for a while, then she closed her eyes and let her head fall back again. "Then tonight is the night you've been looking for," she said very calmly. "I'll hang here all night and you can whip me to a fucking bloody mess! But but there is no goddamn way you're going to break me tonight. No goddamn way!"

She took a deep breath. "Take your best shot," she finished. "You'll never have a better chance."

I chickened out. I left her hanging there for a while until I finished the brandy, then I whipped her again briefly. I knew that she was in a lot of pain but she never even whimpered.

So I took her down and took her to bed.

"No guts?" Vanessa asked after we were in bed.

"I decided that I'd rather have you blow me all night like you promised," I explained.

"Tough shit, loser," Vanessa growled at me. "You chickened out. You eat me first."

What the hell. She was right, of course.

On several occasions I arranged to give Vanessa the chance to dominate a submissive male. The first time I did that she went out and bought herself a very long, thin, steel-cored English riding whip, and that became her favorite instrument for punishment because she could control it so much better than the kind of flexible whips that I usually use.

True to her expressed fantasy, the bigger they were the better she liked them, because no matter how long it took, she would keep at it until her subject literally begged for mercy. And the longer it took, the more fun she had. But that didn't end the torment—just the physical part. Vanessa invented a very special postscript for these sessions that involved a rather cruelly calculated form of psychological torture.

Very simply, after she had "broken" her victim, Vanessa would strip naked and allow me to tie her face-to-face with the man she had just finished whipping. I would tie her wrists to the same rings that his were tied to and tie her ankles to his ankles. Then I would pass a strap around their waists and pull it tight, forcing them to press their bodies against each other. And then I'd take that same riding whip and begin to use it on Vanessa. With each stroke Vanessa's body would involuntary jerk and grind against the body of her "slave," but she would never scream. Instead, she would keep up a steady commentary designed to add to the man's humiliation.

She'd say things like, "He's whipping me much harder than I whipped you, but I'm not screaming like you did"; or, "I only weigh 105 pounds and you weigh over 200, but I can take more than you did"; or, "John's a *real* man—that's why I let him dominate me. But a sniveling weakling like you could never even hope to have a woman like me"; or, "Harder, John! Let's show this miserable shit of a slave what a *real* woman is made of!"

Later I would untie Vanessa, leaving the submissive male still tied, and I would take Vanessa and make violent love to her on the couch in front of him, letting him watch us helplessly. It was quite a scene, and Vanessa loved doing it.

And what always blew my mind was that those poor male "slaves" always wanted to come back to see Vanessa again.

But Vanessa never let them.

I still see Vanessa today, although now we live far apart so it isn't too often. But she has been a steady partner of mine in several memorable episodes.

Vanessa has never changed. She is still the consummate "challenger." I got a fiftieth birthday card from her recently with a note enclosed. It said:

Now that you've reached the mid-century mark, I rather doubt that you'll ever again be of much use to me. After all, there's no 50-year-old man alive who could make me say "please." But if you'd like one more chance, let me know. I'll warm some milk, get out the whips, and try not to yawn.

She was asking for it.
She got it!

9

Karen
(My First "O")

Excerpt from a letter from Karen

There is no way that I can tell you how much I love you. Maybe that's because I have never before felt this way about any man and therefore I have never learned the right words to say.

I was perfectly happy being the person I was before you entered my life. I had everything I'd ever wanted. But then you came along, and suddenly there is a whole new world that I never knew about and now I have to be part of that world or I will die.

You give me so much, every day, and sometimes I feel so inadequate in my ability to give back to you in return . . . to offer you something that will tell you how much I love you. But I don't know what that could be, because there is nothing I can think of with a value that matches what I feel for you. So please, my love, if there is anything I can give you, no matter what the cost, please tell me and let me know the marvelous happiness that will be mine when I bring that gift to you.

I have had three virgins in my life. One of them was Karen.

I don't think that being the first man to sleep with a woman is any great achievement. But in this case I think it helps explain what made Karen my first "O."

It didn't start that way. As a matter of fact, I first dated Karen's roommate, Joyce, for almost a year and when it became obvious that Joyce and I were sleeping together, Karen immediately disapproved.

Karen was then twenty-five years old. She had short, dark, curly hair; a pretty face; dark eyes; a lovely smile; and a small but absolutely beautiful body . . . maybe 5′ 2″ with good legs, a flat hard belly, and sensationally full firm breasts that really didn't need a bra, although she always wore one.

But despite her very good looks, Karen was a convinced Catholic and a devout Virgin—most definitely with a capital V—and so she was very uncomfortable about the fact that Joyce and I were sleeping together. When she found out that I was a married man, that just compounded her disapproval, and she really disliked me intensely at first.

Joyce had a job that required her to leave for work at eight in the morning, while Karen had a job with a production unit at CBS and her hours were ten to six. And so every once in a while, after Joyce had left for work, Karen and I would have breakfast together at their apartment, where we would talk about all sorts of things. I'm a pretty good talker, and little by little Karen decided that she could accept me—and eventually she even got to like me. Then one morning Karen woke up feeling sick, so I fixed her some breakfast and sat with her while she ate it in bed. Then I gave her a back rub. Karen later told me that that was the first time a man's hands had ever touched her body anywhere except on her face or arms. Two weeks later, I gave Karen another back rub just because she liked it, and that morning she hugged me and kissed me goodbye on the cheek.

A few weeks after that, Joyce and I broke up, and the very next night I took Karen to dinner, mainly to sing the blues. Instead we just had a good time with each other, and that's when it really all began. It started very slowly, but in what I like to think was the best possible way. First we fell in love. Karen knew I was married and knew that I also loved my wife very much. But I also sincerely loved Karen and she loved me back—totally. And only after we fell in love did we begin any form of sexual involvement.

We didn't kiss goodnight until our third date. Two weeks later Karen opened her mouth when I kissed her. After maybe two months she allowed me to put my hand on her breast, over her clothes of course, and then, a few weeks later, she allowed my hand under her clothes. Finally, after almost four months, we lay together in the same bed, both completely naked, and my fingers gave Karen her very first orgasm.

After that, Karen knew that she wanted to make love to me "all the way," but it took a while. She frequently masturbated me while I used my fingers and tongue to give her numerous orgasms. However, I had promised her that I wouldn't force her to join me in actual intercourse until she was completely ready. I kept that promise, but it wasn't easy.

Karen began "testing" herself. And me. She would take top and put my cock partway into her, moving her body down slowly until she could feel my erection pressing against her still unbroken hymen, and then she would move very slowly and very carefully up and down until she climaxed. Finally she would kneel next to me and jerk me off. For her it was great. For me it was something else.

Finally, one night we went to bed, and Karen and I caressed and kissed and held each other for a long time as we usually did. Then Karen gently pushed me onto my back and took her customary top position. She eased my cock partway into her and began her gentle pumping. She had her hands on my chest to help balance herself, while her fingers were playing gently with my nipples, just as mine did with hers.

After several minutes Karen carefully leaned forward and kissed me, her tongue teasing the inside of my mouth, and then she straightened up again. She stopped moving and just looked at me for a minute. Then she closed her eyes, took a deep breath, and I heard her whisper, "I love you so much!"

Then Karen raised her body and brought it down again, hard, driving my cock all the way into her.

And she screamed!

Immediately I reached up to take Karen by the shoulders and, without withdrawing my cock, I rolled both of us over so that I was on top of her, keeping my upper body raised with my arms. Then I fucked her, not roughly but very slowly and very gently, easing my cock back so that just the tip was inside her and then slowly sliding it back into her again as deep as I could make it go. I lasted a long time—maybe as many as two hundred strokes—and all the time Karen lay under me quietly, barely moving, her eyes closed and her hands resting lightly on my shoulders as my body moved inside hers.

I came finally and bent to kiss Karen's breasts, and then I lowered my body so that its full length was touching hers; Karen put her arms around me and hugged me. We lay that way quietly for a while, and then she pushed me back gently so that she could look at me. She just stared at me for a couple of minutes, looking very serious, but at last she spoke. "Now I belong to you completely," she whispered. "My mind has been yours for a long time, but now you own my body, too. And my soul."

We made love again early in the morning and it was very good for both of us. But later, when I came back from the bathroom after taking a shower, I found Karen, sitting on one side of the bed, staring at a very large blood stain, and crying. I knelt next to her and held her gently in my arms, not saying anything. Finally Karen stopped crying and turned to me. She sniffled and wiped at her tears with the back of one hand, and then she sort of half smiled.

"I'm OK," she said. "At least one reason I was crying was because I waited so long."

After that our affair was total. Karen and I spent every minute together that we could. I stayed with her at least two nights a week, and when I couldn't stay over we would at least spend an hour or so together after work; or else I would come into the city early to be with her before she went to work. And we spent at least two lunch hours together each week.

We made love constantly. I had thought that I was slowing down —after all, I over was over thirty years old, which isn't exactly over the hill but it isn't like being like a teenager, either. But with Karen I was like a kid. Sometimes we kept score, and one night, between 7:00 P.M. and nine the next morning, we actually made love ten times, and I climaxed during seven of them!

Karen climaxed fourteen times!

She had no inhibitions left at all. We tried every position we'd ever heard of and then invented some of our own. We fucked in the shower. She jerked me off in a movie and another time she did the same thing in a restaurant. She became an expert at oral sex, and when I arranged to take her on a business trip she blew me on a night flight to Atlanta.

Best of all, it seemed as if we were always laughing.

For the first time ever I thought about leaving my wife and asking Karen to marry me. One night, in a sort of roundabout way, I told Karen what I had been thinking of. "No way!" Karen said very firmly. "You're the first and only man I've ever loved and maybe you'll be the only one I'll ever love in my whole life, but if you left your wife and kids for me I wouldn't be able to handle it. I'd have to leave you." She made it quite clear that she meant it.

The letter I quoted above was written on the 3-month anniversary of the night Karen had stopped being a virgin, but instead of mailing the letter she brought it to me when we met for dinner at the old New York Gaslight Club. I read it while we were waiting for dinner and I read it again while we were having after-dinner brandies.

"It's the most beautiful letter anyone ever wrote me," I said to her.

"I mean every word of it," she said. "Please tell me what I can give you."

"There isn't anything," I told her.

"There must be," she insisted. "Maybe not a physical thing like a car or something. Besides, I don't have that kind of money. But maybe something from my heart." She took my hand. "You're the only man I've ever made love to in my life and I've only been doing it for three months, so everything we do together is new to me. I wish there were something I could give you that would be new for you, too, but all I know about sex is what you've taught me."

"It's new for me, too," I told her, and I meant it. "Maybe not the things we do but the way we love each other makes them feel different. And we have done some things that I've never done with anyone else."

"How about the other way around?" Karen asked. "There must be things you've done with other women that you haven't done with me, aren't there?"

I hesitated. "Oh, I suppose so, I guess."

Karen jumped on it. "Like what? Tell me!"

What the hell, I thought. "I've tied girls up and made love to them," I told her.

Karen didn't even blink. "Anything else?"

"I've also tied girls up and whipped them."

Karen took a sip of her brandy this time. "Did you enjoy doing that?" she asked.

I nodded my head. "Very much. And then I added, "So did they."

"Please tell me about it," Karen begged.

As best I could, I explained the pleasures I'd gotten from S/M. I told her about Carol. I tried to explain the thrill and excitement and feeling of power and incredible sexual highs that I got from the domination of a woman. When I finally finished, Karen asked me one more question: "Would you like to have me that way?"

I couldn't lie to her. "I would rather have you as a slave than any other woman in the world."

Karen took my hand and smiled. "Then that's my gift, love," she said. "No matter what you want from a woman, I want to be the one to give it to you. Anything at all. No limits, no exceptions. Friend, lover, whore, or slave, I want to be every kind of woman you've ever had or ever wanted." She paused and squeezed my hand. "Just one other thing," she continued. "I want you to tell me every detail of everything you ever did to every girl you've ever had as a slave."

"Why?"

"Because no matter what you ever did to them—no matter how long you whipped them or how hard you whipped them—I want to know that you have whipped me harder and longer." She looked up at me. "Please promise me that you will do that for me."

"Are you sure that's what you want?" I asked.

There was absolutely no hesitation. "I've never been more sure of anything in my life," Karen said.

"Then I promise," I told her.

Eventually, I kept that promise.

That night, however, I tied Karen to her bed and whipped her gently. Then I untied her and made love to her. When I woke up the next morning, I discovered Karen kneeling naked next to the bed. Her ankles were tied together and her hands were also tied together in front of her. Her head was bowed and there was a small cardboard sign hung around her neck.

The sign read, "SLAVE."

We didn't go to work that day. Instead we spent the entire day and all that night exploring this new relationship. I kept Karen in some form of bondage the entire time. I had Karen bathe me and then rewash every square inch of my body with her tongue while her hands were kept tied behind her. I tied her over the back of a chair and alternately spanked her and fucked her for a very long time.

I ordered her to call me "Sir" at all times. I had her kneel next to me whenever there was nothing else happening, which she did for nearly an hour while I read the paper and did the crossword puzzle.

In the afternoon I "hogtied" Karen with her hands tied behind her and then tied to her bound ankles. I left her that way in a closet while I went shopping for supper, and after she had cooked supper I had her kneel next to me while I ate. Her hands were tied behind her again, and I fed her with my fingers.

She washed the dishes with clothespins on her nipples and when at last she told me that they hurt, I ordered her to leave them on while she scrubbed the kitchen floor. After she finished, I allowed her to remove the clothespins from her breasts and I inspected the floor. I, of course, found places that weren't clean enough, so she had to put the clothespins back on her nipples and do the floor over again. Twice.

Later Karen made love to me with her hands tied behind her, using her mouth at first and then taking top, using only the muscles in her legs to ride up and down on my cock until I had my orgasm.

Finally I tied her upright to the door of her bedroom closet, whipped her once more briefly but quite hard, and then went to bed, intending to leave her there all night. She never made a sound after I'd gone to bed but I couldn't sleep. Besides, I was lonely. So after perhaps an hour and a half I got up, untied her, and took her to bed with me. I retied her hands over her head to a corner of the bed and this time I made love to her, bringing her to orgasm first with my hand, and then again with my tongue, and a third time with my cock. Then I went to sleep, holding her tight to me.

But before I went to sleep I heard Karen whisper, "Good night, Sir. Your slave loves you."

Being my total slave obsessed Karen. She called me "Sir" or "Master" routinely, while I called her "slave." She would kiss my hand whenever we met in public and in private she would kneel and kiss my feet. She knelt next to me whenever I sat down, and began asking my permission to perform even the most routine acts. She bought two harem costumes in a store near Times Square and wore them whenever we were at home alone. I bought her a studded collar, which she wore at home, too, and sometimes in public.

I had a silver ankle chain made for her with the word "slave" engraved on it, and once I had put it on her she never took it off.

I had a key to her apartment, of course, and if I got there after she did I would usually find her kneeling just inside the door, waiting for me. Sometimes she would have tied or chained herself in some way, and often she would have put clamps on her nipples.

One time I found her kneeling, naked and gagged, her hands handcuffed behind her. On the cocktail table in front of her was a note. It read, "Sir: Please whip me fifty times before you remove the gag. I'll explain why later."

I whipped her back as she knelt there, and although she was crying by the time I finished, she never moved or tried to get away from the whip. After the final lash I removed the gag and the handcuffs.

"Thank you, Sir," she whispered, still crying.

"You're welcome. Now how about the explanation?"

Karen wiped her eyes with her knuckles, then looked up at me and sort of laughed. "I just felt so damn happy all day," she said, "that I wanted to share it with you." Then she reached out and hugged me around the knees. "God, I love you!" she said, almost fiercely.

"You're an asshole, slave," I told her.

"Anything you say, Sir," she answered.

Three months after Karen had become my slave, I rented the apartment in Soho. We had decided that we wanted some place other than her apartment that we could equip specially for our Master-slave relationship. Karen helped me look for a suitable place. One of the criteria we had established was that it had to have high ceilings because Karen wanted to experience suspension, being hung by her wrists or ankles. Finally we found what we were looking for: a little studio apartment in an older building that cost only $100 a month. It was even furnished.

The first thing I did was install suspension rings in the ceiling. Karen hung my cat-o'-nine-tails over the head of the bed. I also installed a ring in the floor next to the bed where Karen would sometimes sleep, chained to that ring.

Shortly after the apartment was ready, Karen asked me to meet her there after work. She also asked me if I would please not get there until after 7:30 and to ring the street bell before coming upstairs and letting myself in.

I did as she asked. When I came in there was a single candle burning in a holder on the table. Karen was naked, gagged, and blindfolded. Her ankles were chained together and there were clamps on her nipples. And she was hanging by her wrists. The chair on which she had stood was lying on its side on the floor behind her, where it had fallen when she kicked it over after hearing the bell.

Later that night I asked her what would have happened if someone else had rung the bell by mistake and I had been delayed.

"Did it please you to find me that way, Sir?" Karen asked.

"Very much, slave."

"Then, what difference would it have made? I still would have been there."

How could I answer that?

Another dimension was slowly added to our relationship. Karen had constantly made me the "gift" of her total submission in private. Now she wanted others to know that she was my slave. One evening I tied Karen up and left her standing naked, with her arms held over her head by chains that ran from her wrists to the ceiling rings. And there I left her for the entire evening while I and three male friends, suitably forewarned, played poker.

By this time we had made friends with other people in the S/M scene. On several occasions, handcuffed and wearing her harem pants but naked to the waist, Karen served cocktails and dinner to me and one or two other couples. Another time I chained her to the ceiling rings, gagged and blindfolded her, and then went across the street to give the keys to the apartment to a trusted fellow dominant, who went back, whipped Karen for about half an hour, and then left again, never saying a word to her. She never knew who it was.

Total immersion came on the evening that Karen, completely naked, crawled on her hands and knees to each of four other men in turn, carrying a riding crop in her teeth and performing fellatio on each while he whipped her.

We went on this way for almost a year and a half, and during that time we shared an intense and total Master-slave relationship.

But then Karen's father, who lived in Tampa, went into the hospital, terminally ill with cancer. Taking a leave of absence from CBS, Karen went to Tampa to help her mother care for him.

He died nine weeks later, and when Karen came back to New York it was all over. She had gone to church to pray for her father, and then gone to confession where she spent almost two hours telling a young priest about our affair. He asked her to come to confession every day for the next two weeks and to attend mass daily. After the two weeks had passed, he asked Karen to give him her "slave" ankle chain, which she had done.

By the time Karen came back, it was as if none of what we had done together had ever happened. She even looked different—no make-up, a severe hairstyle, and conservative clothes. We saw each other just once more, meeting in a restaurant for dinner.

"I'm a virgin again, John," Karen told me. She explained that the Catholic Church had taken her back, and that in her new "spiritual identity," our relationship had never happened in the eyes of God.

After dinner Karen shook my hand, told me she would pray for me, said goodbye, and walked out. I never saw her again.

Her father had left her a little money, so Karen quit her job and moved back to Tampa, where she got a job at a local radio station. Two years later I heard that she had gotten married, and several years ago I heard that she had four children.

I hope she's happy.

I still love her.

10

Early Lessons

In S/M, as in everything else, there's a lot to learn.

I was lucky because I learned a lot of very important lessons early, and from some pretty special people who weren't really trying to teach me anything.

LESSON ONE

Excerpt from a letter from Mary L____

There's one way to make sure you're never diasappointed in bed, and that is to never go to bed with anyone you wouldn't want to go to the movies with.

That's pretty good advice. I got it from Mary L____, a white ex-hooker married to a black piano player who worked in a small New York bar. Mary was ten to fifteen years older than I, and she wrote me that letter after I'd sat with her for several hours one evening talking about some unhappy affair.

It was good advice, and it applies to S/M, too. "Never have any-one as a slave that you wouldn't want to have as a friend."

One of the more common activities in the S/M scene involves what's called "humiliation," in which self-proclaimed "Masters" deliberately humiliate their "slaves" either verbally or physically, calling them names such as "filth" or "cunt," possibly urinating on them, and so on.

For many, this is a turn-on, and the submissive recipients of this kind of abuse must get some sort of fulfillment from such mistreatment. But for me it is a big zero. If I am going to have a woman for a "slave," I want to be *proud* of her. Just as important—maybe more— I want her to be proud of *herself.* In my mind the "dominant" and "submissive" roles have nothing to do with the individuals' worth as human beings, and it takes just as much strength and conviction to be a "slave" as it does to be a "Master."

So to me the ultimate thrill and pleasure is having a truly classy woman decide to give herself to me in submission . . . not because she feels that she is of any less value, but simply because that is the role she chooses for her own fulfillment.

In short, first give me a woman who is good enough to be anything she wants to be. Then let me be good enough to make her want to be my slave!

LESSON TWO

A Master *must* experience pain.

When a Master whips a slave he should know what that slave feels.

There are two reasons for this. The first is practical. A Master has the right and the power to inflict pain on his slave. Often the slave is bound and sometimes gagged. Under such conditions there is no limit to the amount of pain or punishment except the judgment and will of the Master. This is as it should be. But if the Master doesn't know what the slave is enduring, if he doesn't know exactly how much pain he is inflicting and how much suffering he is causing, then he may go too far.

Or not far enough.

There is an important psychological reason, too. If a Master knows exactly what his slave is feeling, then his pleasure and satisfaction are so much greater. If he has experienced the feel of a particular whip on his own body, how much more exciting it is to watch that same whip bite into the naked body of his slave, while knowing exactly what kind of pain it is that the slave is experiencing.

But I learned an ever bigger lesson years ago from a young lady in Birmingham, Alabama. Her name was Odette and she was a waitress in a local steak house. I was then traveling to Birmingham about once a month, staying two or three days on each visit. I had taken Odette home one evening after she had waited on me, and we had thoroughly enjoyed each other.

After that I saw Odette every time I went to Birmingham, and on one of our early dates I told her about some of my S/M adventures. She was turned on by the stories, so that night I tied her to the closet door in my hotel room and whipped her. It was exciting for both of us, but Odette immediately decided that some day she wanted to try the other role. She wanted to see what it would be like to whip *me*.

There used to be a motel near the Birmingham Airport, where half the rooms, either all the even-numbered rooms or all the odd-numbered ones, have cathedral ceilings with exposed wooden beams. That's where Odette and I always stayed when I was in town. I often used those beams to tie Odette and sometimes, when I was feeling mean, to suspend her in preparation for a whipping.

As our sessions progressed, Odette became able to handle increasingly severe levels of discipline and find them sexually exciting, but she still wanted very much to have the chance to "turn the tables" on me and eventually I had to resort to dirty tricks. Before each session we'd flip a coin, and whoever won would get to choose who would be the "Master." The dirty trick was that, as an amateur magician, I can make a coin come up any way I want it to, so of course Odette always lost. She was good-natured about it. Being dominated was a kick for her and, besides, the whippings and other torments that I imposed on her were carefully controlled and definitely heightened her sexual pleasure and performance.

But Odette was still frustrated. "Shit!" I remember her saying one night as the coin came up my way again. "That's six fucking times in a row you've won!" She sighed and smiled at me. "Sooner or later, big boy," she said. "Sooner or later you're going to get yours."

"Sooner or later," I agreed as I began the process of tying Odette, but I was mentally crossing my fingers.

But I screwed up. That simple. One night when she called "tails," I lost my concentration and tails it was.

"Hot damn!" Odette yelled.

"Oh, shit!" I said to myself.

I couldn't bring myself to chicken out. I didn't want to be whipped, but reneging on the deal would have been even worse, so I gritted my teeth, smiled bravely, and turned myself over to the very eager young lady.

I had taught Odette how to use padding if you were going to suspend someone, and she did that first, wrapping a hand towel around my wrists before tying a rope to each one. Then she asked me to strip and had me stand on the cocktail table while she passed the two ropes over one of the beams, stretching my arms tightly before tying the knots. Finally she took one more piece of rope and tied my ankles together.

Odette was ready. Boy, was she ready! She took my belt and stood in front of me so she could look at me. "I want you to help me," she said. "I've never done this before so I don't know how far I should go. So I want you to do me a favor. I'm going to whip you with the belt like you've whipped me and I'm asking you to take as much as you possibly can. I want to see how much that is. I hope it's a lot. But when you finally reach your limit—when you just can't take anymore—then tell me." Then Odette smiled at me.

"But I want you to tell me in a special way," she told me. "When you can't take any more I want you to step off the table so that you're hanging by your wrists. I know what that feels like, and I know it will be hard for you. That's why I picked that way for you to let me know when you've had it, because I know you won't want to do it, so maybe you'll really push yourself."

I couldn't help wondering how long Odette had been thinking about this night. She seemed to have it pretty well planned. Odette looked me right in the eye. "Will you do that for me?" she asked. "Will you really try for me?"

I guess I felt guilty or something, but right then I decided to give her the best I had—that she deserved as much as I could give her. "You're on," I told her. "I'll hang in as long as I can. Have a good time."

"Oh, you bet your ass I will!" Odette answered, and she began the whipping.

She was a little awkward at first, but she seemed to get the feel of it. Before long the belt was cutting into my back and legs and chest and belly, leaving a wide red mark each time it hit me. Odette was pretty good. She kept walking around and around me, picking a different target for each stroke, and keeping a slow methodical pace.

And all the time she was talking softly. "Oh, I love it!" she would say in a half whisper. "Oh, God, I love it! Don't quit, baby. Please don't quit! You can have me the next time, and we won't even flip the coin. But don't quit on me. Take it for me, honey. Please take it for me!"

I guess it was a matter of pride. I gritted my teeth and hung in. My body flinched involuntarily at almost every stroke, and once in a while she'd hit me extra hard or the belt would wrap around my body so that the tip would cut into me; or maybe it would catch a place that had already been hit several times before, and at these times I'd cry out a little. But I let her keep going, and I even turned my head and bit my own shoulder for a while. But finally, of course, I just couldn't handle any more and so I took a deep breath, picked up my feet, and allowed myself to swing clear of the cocktail table, giving Odette the signal she had asked for.

Immediately Odette pulled the cocktail table away and then she came back and stood in front of me again. "Thanks, baby," she said. "You really tried for me." She paused and I hung there, waiting for her to put the table back.

"That was one hundred and sixty-seven," she told me. "I kept count." And then she let me have it. "Those were for you, baby," she said. "The next one hundred and sixty-seven are for *me*."

She really did it! I hung there by my wrists while Odette did it all over again! I couldn't believe she was actually doing it. I'd taken as much as I possibly could and now it was going to happen again, but so much worse, because now the pain of the belt, striking my already agonized body, would be compounded by the pain of being suspended by my wrists.

I tried not to scream, but I know I did with each lash. Somehow, though, I managed not to beg.

It was total torture. Before Odette began the second whipping I had already forced myself to go to what I thought were my absolute limits. Now, with the pain even greater than before, I was totally beyond those limits. Through the terrible agony I heard Odette counting the strokes. I knew that she was actually going to go all the the way and I knew that I couldn't possibly endure it.

But halfway through, just as I was about to break and beg her to stop, something very strange happened. It's hard to describe, but it was suddenly as if I had become two people. One of those people was hanging there being whipped while the other was sort of off to one side, watching, and somehow my mind moved to that second person. I was still in very great pain but for the rest of the whipping I just hung there quietly and let it happen, almost giving my body to the belt and the pain, and I think in that state I could have taken even more than Odette gave me.

Since that time I've heard submissives describe the same thing—of being forced to endure torment beyond any previous limits. "It's like going over a cliff," one told me. "One minute the pain is so bad you want to die and the next minute it's like it's happening to someone else."

It was a terribly painful lesson. I know that I'd never have the courage to try it again. But I'm still glad that I was forced to go through it once, because now I know what truly *total* pain is.

More important, it taught me that under very special circumstances a submissive can be taken beyond her conceived limits, and I know what she is feeling when that happens. It has to be done very carefully, and you have to know exactly what to look for and what the ultimate limits are. But it can be done.

Done right, it is one of the greatest feelings of dominance and power and fulfillment that a Master can possibly have.

As for the slave, she will always remember it . . . and if you have picked the right one, she will remember it with tremendous pride!

LESSON THREE

Excerpt from a letter from Martha

. . . *So when you come to Savannah again, please try to work it so we can have four days together. There are so many things that I want to do for you and with you and to you.*

I want to do my "Dance of the Seven Veils" for you. (I take off eight.)

I want to strip us both naked to the waist and dance with you, holding you very close, and see how long we can dance before one of us drags the other to the bed.

I want to show you that I can make love to you in a way that feels so good that you'll beg me to stop.

That didn't sound all bad. Martha was a lovely red-haired Southern belle. She was ten years older than I and very pretty, very sensual, and very wise.

Separated from her husband in Atlanta, Martha and her two young sons were living with her elderly aunt. Martha was working as a receptionist at a company I called on; when I asked her to dinner, Martha promptly invited me to come home with her and "meet the family." A month later I arranged to stop over in Savannah again for a weekend, and on the second night Martha stayed with me at my hotel. It was very good.

Martha later explained that Savannah was a "real small town" and for that reason having an affair was difficult. She loved making love, she told me, but it had been six months since the last time. I told her I was sorry for her but glad for me.

We traded letters and we dated again a few weeks later when I managed to be in Savannah for just one night. Again it was beautiful— ten hours of almost non-stop love-making—and it was after that visit that Martha told me in that same letter I quoted above:

I can make love to you in a way that will feel so good that you'll beg me to stop.

That I had to see.

I did.

I arranged for a long weekend about two months later, arriving in Savannah Thursday night. We were like kids. We went to dinner and then back to my hotel suite where we tried her "challenge dance." Martha stripped herself to the waist and then, insisting that I keep my hands at my sides, she slowly stripped me of my jacket, tie, and shirt. Then she kicked off her shoes, found some quiet music on the radio, and we danced.

Sometimes her body was pressed tightly against mine, her breasts and belly flattened against me. At other times she pulled back so that only our hands were touching each other, so that I could just look at her and study the excitement of her lovely body. Best of all was when she would dance close enough so that just the tips of her breasts touched my chest and she'd move her body slowly, stroking me with her hardened nipples while her fingers played with the back of my neck.

It went on that way for almost an hour, and later we decided to call it a draw.

The next night we took champagne and a picnic basket to the coast and made love on the beach by the ocean.

Saturday night we went to a party and didn't get home until four in the morning.

On Sunday morning we took her kids and aunt to church; finally, that afternoon, I asked Martha about her letter.

"I meant it," she said. "I can do something to you that's so doggone sexy that you'll beg me to stop. It won't hurt—it will just feel so good that you won't be able to stand it."

"You're going to have to prove it." I told her.

"My pleasure," Martha said, "but you're going to have to let me tie you up."

That threw me. I wasn't at all sure about letting anyone tie me up, even if it was only so they could make love to me. But Martha teased and kidded and pouted until, finally, I gave in. She tied me spread-eagle, face up on the bed, using two of my neckties and two of her cloth belts. I was naked, of course.

Next she used her hand and mouth to bring me to erection. It didn't take long.

And then she went to work.

Fox fur neckpieces were then fashionable and Martha had worn hers to church that morning. She went to get it, then knelt between my legs and draped the fur around my cock. "Hang on," she warned me, and, holding one end of the long fur piece in each hand, she pulled it towards her until it was taut around my rock-hard penis. Then, very slowly and very gently, she began teasing my cock with the fur, using the same sort of "polishing" motion as a shoe shine boy would with a polishing cloth. Back and forth . . . back and forth . . .very slowly while she just knelt there between my legs and smiled at me.

For about two minutes I felt marvelous. Then I began feeling like I was just about ready to come, but I couldn't. And after maybe four minutes at the very most, my cock was so incredibly sensitive that I thought I was going to go crazy.

Martha was right. It didn't hurt. It just felt so unbelievably good that I couldn't stand it.

"You win," I told her, almost gasping.

Martha smiled. "No, John, darling, *you* win," and she just knelt there and smiled at me while she kept the fur piece moving on my cock.

I fought the bindings. I arched my body and twisted back and forth. I begged her to stop.

"When I'm ready," Martha told me. She was obviously having a ball!

Finally, when I started to scream, Martha gave in. She suddenly speeded up her motions, doing it very fast, maybe eight or ten times while I kept screaming. And then she dropped the fur piece on the floor and moved to straddle me. "I think you're ready for me now," she whispered as she slowly lowered herself to take me inside her. She was soaking wet and my cock slid into her with no effort. God, it felt good! Then Martha rode me very slowly, moving her body up and down while she played with her own nipples.

When I came, I screamed again.

So "torture" doesn't have to involve pain, and it works for women, too. On many occasions I've carried out this kind of sensual torture on female submissives, tying them first and then slowly and carefully bringing them to orgasm or to the very brink of orgasm, and then "held" them there, right at the peak of that sensation, sometimes for as long as twenty or even thirty minutes!

And women scream, too.

It doesn't work for all women, but when it does it is tremendously exciting.

For *both* of us.

LESSON FOUR

Excerpt from a note from Gretchen

The kind of dominant I'm looking for is the kind who can control me totally with just one word, or simply a look. That's hard to find, but I'm a quality submissive and I deserve a quality Master.

Perhaps the most important early lesson that I ever learned was that a *real* Master doesn't need a chain or a whip. He simply has to believe in himself.

That note was written by a lovely lady named Gretchen, whom I only saw five times over a period of some two and a half years, but who literally bombarded me with a series of notes and letters that I finally dubbed "submissive thought for the week."

But unlike a lot of heavy-duty correspondents who chicken out in a real face-to-face meeting, Gretchen put her mind and her body behind her written words. Gretchen was a stewardess. Since she was based on the West Coast and I was living in New York, our meetings were rare. I first met her on a flight, but not one she was working. Instead, she was "dead-heading" back to her home near Los Angeles; by luck the last seat on the flight, assigned to Gretchen at the last minute, was next to mine.

There's something about planes that causes people to talk freely (Ships are even better that way—or worse, depending on your viewpoint.) Anyway, by the time the crew was serving dinner, Gretchen and I had each other pretty well pegged.

I think it started when I was telling Gretchen some story which she interrupted. Without even thinking, I said, "quiet" rather sternly, and Gretchen immediately shut up and allowed me to finish. At the time I didn't even realize what I'd done, but after I stopped talking Gretchen just looked at me for quite a while before she finally said, "May I have permission to speak, Sir?"

At first I thought Gretchen was kidding and I laughed at her, but then I realized that she was quite serious. "You don't need my permission," I told her.

"You told me to be quiet a few minutes ago," Gretchen explained, "and the way you said it left little doubt in my mind that I'd better do whatever you say."

Now it was my turn to study her. "Are you always so obedient?" I asked her at last.

"I prefer the word 'submissive,' Sir," Gretchen answered.

That, of course, took care of that. By the time the plane landed in Los Angeles we had, without ever really trying, established a fully matured dominant/submissive relationship with each other. Gretchen referred to me as "Sir" routinely and with total naturalness. She responded instantly to deliberately trivial orders, such as sitting with her hands folded in her lap, putting cream and sugar in my coffee for me, or asking the stewardess to bring me another drink. She even asked my permission to go to the bathroom, keeping her eyes downcast, not looking at my face. And when we parted at the airport, having made a date for the following evening, I extended my hand, which she took and kissed.

I called Gretchen late the next afternoon and gave her some very explicit instructions regarding how I expected her to act when I came to her apartment that evening, and she obeyed completely. When I rang at the lobby door and identified myself, Gretchen "buzzed" me into the building. When I arrived at her apartment door, I found it unlocked. Letting myself in, I found Gretchen exactly as I had instructed, dressed only in a black garter belt and black stockings, kneeling in the middle of the living room, her back straight, her hands resting on her well-spread thighs, her head thrown back, her eyes closed, and her mouth partly open. There was a riding crop on the floor next to her.

Gretchen had, as ordered, left out a chilled bottle of white wine and glasses. I had brought a newspaper, so I poured myself some wine, settled on the sofa, and began to read the paper, deliberately taking my time. Even though I stretched it out for close to an hour, Gretchen never moved. When I finally "released" her from this position, she crawled to me, kissed my hand, and sat on the floor by my feet.

Later that evening I ordered Gretchen to stand spread-eagled facing the living room wall, arms stretched high and legs well apart. I told her that, even without actual ropes, she was to consider herself "tied" and that I did not expect her to move. Then I took the riding crop and slowly used it to whip her back and bottom and the back of her legs, gently at first, but then quite hard and finally harder still. I know that it hurt her, but although she cried out several times, particularly at the end, she never moved.

It never changed during the few times that I was with Gretchen. During all of the time we spent together she was a totally obedient slave, submissively devoting her mind and her body and her actions to whatever I chose, without questions, without reservations, and without chains.

Of course I still use the chains frequently, but ever since meeting Gretchen I have at one time or another subjected every new relationship with a submissive to this important test of "true mastery." And I have taken great satisfaction and pleasure from achieving total domination of my partner with, as Gretchen put it, "just one word, or simply a look."

11

Margot

Not everyone fits the patterns.

Take Margot.

Margot was a chunky little lady from Montreal, thirty-one years old when we first met, and absolutely unique. She matched none of the "submissive stereotypes" that I'd established for myself. She was strictly one of a kind.

Excerpt from an advertisement

N.Y.C. male with dominant personality and actions to match seeks woman who shares my views of an ordered and disciplined world where men are men and women are expected to love, honor, and obey.

I hate to admit it now, but I was pretty proud of that advertisement when I ran it in *Confidential Flash* some years ago. But it served its purpose and brought me several interesting responses, including one from a six-foot-six black transvestite in Montreal who sent me a picture of him/herself dressed in a tutu together with a long, long letter written on pink perfumed stationary . . . all in poetry.

That one I never answered but I did answer a few, including one deceptively simple postcard.

I saw your ad in C.F. *and I think we might get along. I'll be in New York the first week of April. Why don't we get together for a drink and see where it goes?*

Margot P———
[Montreal Address]

If I'd known exactly where it was going to go over the next three years I'm not sure I would have answered, but I did answer, and once I'd met Margot there was no turning back.

We met on the Thursday of Margot's week-long visit to New York. We had by this time traded a couple of rather nice but noncommittal letters. I had hoped to see her earlier in the week in case things went well, but Margot had already filled most of her schedule with dinner and theater dates with other friends. Besides, it seems that what she had in mind for our get-together was best held off for the end of the week so that she could go home to Montreal afterward and rest.

Margot was staying at the old Barclay Hotel on East 48th Street. We agreed that I'd call her from the lobby after work and that we'd meet in the Gold Room, a lovely cocktail lounge in that hotel that's closed now. I called Margot shortly after 5:00 P.M. and then went to the Gold Room and sat at the bar. I'd gotten into an involved conversation with the bartender when I felt a tap on my shoulder. Turning on my stool, I found myself facing a five-foot-two, slightly stocky version of Bridget Bardot with shoulder-length streaked blonde hair, beautiful green eyes, and a wonderfully friendly smile—all topped off with the slightest hint of a French-Canadian accent. I was so enchanted that I immediately decided to take her to dinner at Le Berry, a tiny restaurant on the West Side where Margot spent three hours babbling happily in French with the family that manned the bar, the kitchen, and the dining room.

After dinner we went down to SoHo for an Irish coffee at a small place near my apartment, where we finally had a chance to compare notes on some of our more basic interests. Margot freely admitted that she thoroughly enjoyed both physical and sexual submission to a truly dominant man, and after some more conversation she made it clear that she felt I fit into that category.

We spent the night together at my apartment and Margot readily agreed to submit to whatever I might choose to subject her to. The only provision she made was that she wanted me to gag her before inflicting any pain. I agreed, although the evening involved only mild levels of discipline, centering instead on some rather intricate forms of enforced sexual and psychological submission. We both enjoyed ourselves immensely, although Margot did tell me later that night, after I had untied her, that she had expected me to be considerably more severe than I had actually been.

The next morning I took Margot back to the Barclay, waited for her to pack, and then took her to brunch at the Carlisle before putting her into a limousine for the ride out to JFK. When we kissed goodbye we both promised that we'd write.

Four months later Margot did—a post card again that said simply, "How have you been?" I wrote back and told her that I'd been fine, and she replied with a "newsy" letter that ended with the hope of spending a long weekend in New York in late summer—a weekend she would very much like to spend with me.

This time I picked Margot up at the airport at about eight in the evening on a Thursday night. Since she had already had dinner on the plane, we went straight down to the apartment in SoHo. I still remembered Margot's comments about me taking it easy that first night, so I had made plans to spend a long evening giving her the chance to see that I could, indeed, be "considerably more severe" than I had been on our first date.

As a matter of fact, on the way downtown I told Margot just that, and her response was simply a nod and a smile.

At the apartment Margot asked that I allow her to take a shower before we started. I gave her permission, using the time to "lay out" some of the equipment I planned to use that night. Margot came out of the shower wrapped in the huge towel I'd given her and stood next to me looking at the various straps, whips, and other implements that I'd arranged on the bed.

"What are you thinking?" I asked her.

Margot continued to stare at the whips. "I'm thinking that I'm going to be in for an interesting evening," she said at last.

I ordered Margot to drop the towel and I began by tying her to a heavy straight-backed armchair, using a number of straps around her arms, legs, waist, and upper body. By the time I finished, Margot was bound so tightly that she could scarcely move a muscle and, at the same time, was completely vulnerable to whatever I might choose to do to her. I was putting the blindfold in place when she finally spoke again. "You are going to use a gag, aren't you?"

"Yes," I told her, adjusting the blindfold.

"Please kiss me before putting it in," Margot asked. I bent to kiss her and then she spoke again. "After you gag me, I want you to look in my purse. There's a letter there for you. Would you please read it before you begin?"

'All right," I agreed.

"Thank you," she said. I kissed her again and then put the leather gag in her mouth, strapping it tightly around her head to hold it securely in place.

Then I went and found the letter.

John,

If everything has gone as I hope it will, I am now bound and gagged and naked and helpless, and I am waiting for you to begin my torture. But before you begin there are some things that I feel you must know.

First, if you look in my little green case, you will find all the letters and postcards you ever sent me. Also my address book. The reason I brought them is so that you will know that there is no trace of you back in Montreal. No one knows where I am or who I am with. That's important because it gives you the freedom to do anything you wish to me without any inhibitions.

Next, I want you to know that I receive no pleasure whatsoever from pain, either physical, mental, or sexual. When you torture me it will be exactly that—torture. But I have to know that the torture is going to happen. That is very important and I want you to know why.

You see, my fulfillment is not in the torture itself as it is with most other submissives. Instead, my fulfillment lies in the marvelously exciting process of talking myself into putting myself in a position in which I will be subjected to torture—of delivering myself to my torturer— of allowing him to render my body totally helpless so that no matter how extreme the tortures are that he has planned, they are, by my own actions, made inevitable.

In addition, it is important for me to know that those tortures will be just that—extreme.

That process, which I have been going through since our last meet-

ing, is now complete. I cannot possibly describe or explain the pleasures I have had in planning this moment and preparing myself for it. So many dreams—so many fantasies—so much excitement—so many beautiful orgasms—all inspired by the slow building of my resolve to deliver myself to you and also by the thoughts and planning of what you will do to me during the next long hours.

Yes, John, I hate the pain, but unless I know that the pain will come—that the tortures will really happen—none of those wonderful pleasures would have been possible for me. It is only when I know in advance that those tortures will really happen and that there will be a point of no return after which I will be utterly helpless to prevent them, and that the person I will be with will be really cruel. Otherwise these marvelous months I have spent preparing for this moment would not have been at all possible.

I know that you are reading this letter and I know what I have written. I ask you now, when I can no longer change my mind, to be cruel—very cruel! The last time we were together you used your whip perhaps fifty times. Why not five hundred? Or five thousand? And why just a whip? What about a crop or a strap? Or think of what your hands or your fists could do to a helpless woman's body.

Do you own a pair of pliers? Think of what they could do to my nipples! Do you have needles? Have you ever wondered what it would feel like to put them under a woman's fingernails? You smoke, but why do you use an ashtray when my body will serve?

Yes, I hate and fear the pain, and I am truly terrified of the torture that I know is about to come. But I must know that it will come or all the rest will have no meaning, and all will have been wasted.

I want you to know that at this moment I am in my own special version of heaven, but soon that heaven will end, its passing probably marked by one final but magnificent orgasm which, based on past experience, will occur with the first stroke of your whip. After that I will be in hell, but you will know that just before that hell began all those months of dreams had at last been totally fulfilled.

So begin, John, and let my agony provide you with equal fulfillment.

Yours,

Margot

Her "agony" lasted five hours that night.

And I *was* fulfilled.

During the next three months I heard nothing from Margot, but one day I got another post card from her. "Been thinking of you," was all the card said. And it started all over again.

Over the next two years that I knew Margot I only saw her four more times. After each meeting I would hear nothing for three or four months, and then I'd get a post card or a letter and the sequence would begin again, slowly building to the incredible climaxes that our actual meetings represented for both of us, although in very different ways.

Each meeting was more extreme than the last, and at times it got scary.

Margot had explained that one of her greatest sources of pleasure resulted from her dreaming up tortures that she could then fantasize actually taking place. She would start while using either her fingers or a vibrator to excite herself sexually while she dreamed up the plot and details of the torture, but she would deliberately delay the climax until all the details of the torture were in place so that she could finally imagine and fantasize the entire act while bringing herself, at last, to orgasm.

But an even greater thrill was possible for her if she knew that she could write down the details of that torture and then arrange for it to actually happen. For that reason she asked me to promise that I would read the notes she brought me and really do these things to her, no matter how extreme they might be. I made her that promise, but again, if I had known where it was going to end, I don't think I would have gone along with her request. But I did make the promise and I did keep it.

It wasn't easy.

In the process of planning her third visit to me in New York Margot asked me to arrange to have forty-eight straight hours available. I found out why when she showed up on Friday afternoon. She brought along a packet of twenty-four envelopes, and at dinner that night she explained that each one contained the details of a different "torture." But it was more complicated than that, because she had made up a whole game to go with those envelopes. She had also brought along two pairs of dice, the idea being that before we began, I would throw all four dice and that the total—which could be anywhere from four to twenty-four—would determine the number of envelopes that would be used and, consequently, the number of "tortures" that she would have to endure during the weekend.

She had also dreamed up variations. For example, after the dice had been thrown and the number determined, I could take that number of envelopes in order. (She had numbered them in a predetermined sequence from numbers one to twenty-four, and she knew what was in each one.) Or I could allow her to pick the right number of envelopes, choosing the ones she really wanted to have carried out. Or I could choose various numbers at random and then perhaps arrange them in some order and give her the list, so that she would know what was to happen.

We didn't use any of these ideas. Instead I dreamed up my own variation. First, while we were waiting for our dessert to be served, I threw the four dice, but in order to heighten the suspense I threw them one at a time. The first one came up a five. The second came up six. Margot commented that she was going to be in for a rough weekend. But then I threw a one and finally a two, so that the total was fourteen. I told her that I planned to shuffle all the envelopes thoroughly, put them all in a box, and then just pick them out one at a time and do whatever each one said until a total of fourteen envelopes had been used.

Margot asked me to tell her which envelope I had picked each time so that she would know what was coming. I told her I'd think about it but that I wouldn't promise. She also asked if she could pick just one envelope of her own choosing and make that the last one. I said that I wouldn't let her do that but, if she wanted, she could pick that one and make it number fifteen. She said she'd think about that.

Finally, Margot pointed out that some of the things she'd planned required her to be bound in some rather elaborate ways. I told her I'd worry about that as we went along. After that Margot just shut up and didn't make any more suggestions or requests. But as we started on our desserts, I could see both the tension and the excitement building in her.

Now that I understood Margot, it was fascinating to observe her as we waited for the time of her ordeal to begin. She was obviously terribly nervous, and I assumed she was very much afraid of what might happen during the weekend. After all, she had taken the primary role in planning our time together and she knew exactly what could happen. But at the same time she was in an extreme state of sexual excitement that was equally obvious. She couldn't sit still. Her nipples showed clearly erect, even through her blouse and bra. I was sure her pussy was soaking wet and I remember thinking that if I so much as touched her on the knee, she would have an orgasm right there in the restaurant.

And so to heighten the suspense, I picked a first envelope at random there in the restaurant and opened it. First, I was curious to see what kind of things Margot had dreamed up. Second, I wanted to know ahead of time what form of bondage I should put Margot in at the start of our session.

The envelope I picked turned out to be number sixteen and I opened it without showing Margot which number it was. Inside was a three-by-five-inch index card. This is what was written on it:

> Roll two dice. Whatever number comes up, hang me by my thumbs for that number of minutes and whip my breasts constantly while I am hanging.

I think I must have looked startled. "Which one did you pick?" Margot asked.

"I'm not sure I'm going to tell you," I answered, "but first you tell me something. How many of those envelopes involve my doing something like rolling the dice again?"

"Oh," Margot said. "You got one of those." She stopped to think for a while, counting on her fingers. "Seven of them have you rolling the dice," she said. "And in four you cut the cards, and in two you flip a coin."

"One other question," I said. "How many of these things you put in the envelopes are things you've really had done to you and how many are things you've only had fantasies about?"

Again Margot stopped to consider before answering. "There are about four that I've experienced pretty much totally," she said at last. "Then there are four or five more that I've come pretty close to. There are another ten or so that I've tried to do to myself but haven't been able to, at least not completely. And the rest are strictly from fantasies. But," she continued, "I'm sure that there's nothing in any of the envelopes that you won't be able to do if you really try."

I studied her for a while. "Which category is number sixteen in?" I asked at last, holding up the index card I'd taken from the envelope.

Margot looked at me and then at the card in my hand and then at me again. Then she took a deep breath. "Hanging by my thumbs," she said in a soft voice, and I saw her look down at her hands in her lap. "I've tried to do that to myself and I almost made it once, but I couldn't quite make myself put all my weight on them." She was still looking at her hands. "But you're really going to do it, aren't you?" she asked in a very quiet voice.

"If you come downtown with me, yes, I am," I told her, "but you can decide to go back to Montreal right now if you want to and I won't stop you."

Margot took another deep breath. "I'll stay with you," she said finally, and then she added, "Just don't forget to gag me before we begin." She was still looking at her hands. "Could we throw the two dice now so I'll know how long it's going to be?" she asked, almost in a whisper.

"No."

"When?" she asked.

"Not until you're actually hanging," I said, "and even then I'm not going to tell you what number comes up on the dice. I won't cheat, but you're going to have to just hang there without knowing how long it's going to be."

That's the way I did it. And I rolled a natural seven.

Some of the other cards I picked that night read:

> Throw one die and multiply by 50. Use the riding crop on me that number of times on any part of my body that you choose.

> Cover both my breasts completely with hot wax dripped from a burning candle. Hold the candle very close to my body.

> Cut the cards. If it's a two through a seven, hang me by my wrists and whip me for 15 minutes. If it's an eight through a king, make it 30 minutes. If it's an ace, make it for an hour, and if it is the Joker, do it for two hours.

> Tie my wrists *behind* my back and then use the hoist to slowly pull me up until I'm *hanging* by them. Leave me there as long as you choose, but whip me all the time while I'm hanging that way.

It was 4:00 in the morning before I had finished the torture detailed on the eighth card. Margot had been gagged the entire time, and her only break had been after the sixth one, when I'd taken her to the bathroom. I decided that we both needed a rest and so I took her to bed, handcuffing one wrist to the frame, and finally removing the gag.

In a choking voice Margot begged me for a glass of water. After drinking it, she curled up into a ball and began to cry. She had, quite literally, been tortured for nearly six hours. What I really expected was for her to beg me to stop it or to let her go home. But she didn't. She simply cried herself to sleep.

Margot was still sleeping when I woke up shortly before noon. I woke her, handcuffed her hands in front of her, took her to the bathroom again, and then brought her another glass of water. She drank it slowly, cupping it with her two chained hands and staring at me over the rim of the glass. Since I'd untied her earlier that morning and put her in bed, the only words she'd spoken were when she'd asked for that first glass of water before going to sleep.

"We still have six envelopes to go," I said to her. She remained quiet, making no response at all. "Do you want me to stop?" I asked next.

Margot looked at me for a long time and she began trembling almost uncontrollably. I waited. Finally she began to talk, her voice shaking: "I wanted you to stop one second after you hung me by my thumbs that first time last night, and that has never changed. It's just gotten worse. It's been horrible . . . all of it . . . and if you unchain me now and leave me alone I will run away. But I know you're not going to let me go and I know that I'm going to be tortured again, and that terrifies me so much that I can't even talk about it." She paused and drank some of the water, her hands shaking so much that she spilled some of it. She was crying when she continued: "But I also know that if you let me go, I will never let myself see you again; but even if you don't stop after six more envelopes but decide to torture me the whole weekend, I know that someday I will come back for even more, and that scares me, too." By now Margot was crying so hard it was difficult to understand her. "Please," she choked out, "don't make me talk anymore. Just do whatever you're going to do."

I finished, just as I had promised her I would. I gagged her again, opened the ninth envelope, and went on with her torture. I took it slowly, however, allowing her time to rest between each card, so it wasn't until early evening that I finally reached into the box and picked the last envelope. It turned out to be number twenty-four:

Hang me by my ankles with my hands chained behind me, and whip
the soles of my feet very hard with your riding crop at least fifty times
on each foot.

I looked at Margot, who was lying tied to the bed where her last torture had required her to be tied. Until now I had not told her in advance
any of the numbers of the envelopes I'd drawn from the box. This
time I decided to tell her but first I untied her, handcuffed her hands
behind her, and allowed her to use the bathroom once more. When
she was ready I picked up the last envelope. "The last envelope is number
twenty-four," I told her.

Margot sat down on the chair next to her, and doubled over so that
her head was on her knees. She began crying again and slowly shaking her head back and forth as if she were saying, "No, no, no, no, no!"

But I went ahead and tied her ankles to a long spreader bar, using
the hoist to hang her clear of the floor and delivering exactly fifty
strokes of the riding crop to each of her feet. Judging by Margot's
reactions, this was one of the most painful tortures of all. I was very
glad when it was finally over.

Margot had planned to go home late Sunday night but something
woke me up about 6:00 that morning; I found her dressed, packed,
and almost ready to leave. "There's a flight this morning at eight o'clock,"
she told me, "and I would like to try to catch it if you'll let me."

I didn't try to stop her, although I think I could have. Instead
I offered to ride out to the airport with her, but she said she'd rather
go alone. So I went downstairs with her, flagged down a taxi, and
said goodbye. I didn't expect to ever see her again.

I was wrong.

Four months later I got another post card, this time from Miami.
"Here for vacation with girlfriend," it said. "Might be in New York
in fall."

I saw Margot twice more. She did come to New York in the fall
and stayed with me for three very rough days. The next summer, I
went to Montreal and stayed with Margot for six days. This was the
time I almost broke my promise and quit on her. Margot had spent
over eight months preparing herself, having written what turned out
to be a twenty-two page detailed scenario for the first four days of
my stay with her, which was originally planned for five days.

Margot was tight as a drum when I arrived, but obviously in a very high state of sexual excitement as well. After all, she had been building up to this for a very long time. As a matter of fact, she was so wound up when I arrived up at her apartment that she couldn't even speak; she simply handed me the outline she'd written, sealed in a manila envelope. On the outside was a note which read: "We begin with me kneeling before you naked, gagged, and blindfolded, my ankles chained together and my hands chained together behind my back and then chained in turn to my ankles."

I hefted the envelope in my right hand, sort of weighing it. "You've done a lot of planning again, it seems," I said. Margot just stared at me and nodded her head. "Well, this time we're going to begin *my* way," I told her. "Now strip!" She did, immediately. I took her right there on the floor of her living room, jamming a pillow under her ass to make it easier for me and fucking her almost mechanically until I'd had my orgasm. All through it Margot clawed at my back and shoulders, screaming as she built to each of four separate, distinct, and tumultuous orgasms of her own before I finally exploded inside her.

Afterward Margot lay on the floor motionless and smiled up at me almost shyly. "Oh, John," she sighed, "that was truly lovely. But now I'm all unwound, damn it!"

"So why don't we forget the script and just fuck for five days?" I suggested.

Margot rolled over and came over to kneel by my feet, putting her head in my lap. "That's so very tempting, love, but I've been working up to this for the better part of a year." She put her arms around my waist and hugged herself to me. "I finished writing that outline three months ago, and since then I've read it to myself almost every night. I've had the most huge and delicious orgasms, and last night I did it one more time and then I didn't sleep all night waiting for you to come this afternoon." She tilted her head back and kissed me. "So if I don't go through with it, it would be such a waste and I might never have the nerve to get ready again." She kissed me once more, long and hard. "But let's not start right now," she whispered. "Let's wait until after dinner, so I can have the time to get myself all wound up again."

We began at ten o'clock that night and didn't finish until early in the morning of the fifth day. During that entire time Margot was in some form of bondage and, except for a few rare, brief intervals, was experiencing at least some pain. She was gagged most of the time, and during the four days she was allowed only some water and a few slices of bread.

The tortures she had planned for the four-day period began modestly but built slowly and steadily in their level of brutality. I cannot possibly describe in detail all of what happened, but it was exhausting even for me and unremitting hell for Margot! During that time, in the process of keeping my promise to her, I did things to Margot that I had never done to another woman before and that I will never, ever do to any other woman again. It was very difficult, and there were several times when I came very close to quitting. (Since that experience I have told people that sometimes it requires as much courage to be a Master as it does to be a slave.)

But I did go all the way; I carried out all of the agonizing torments in Margot's scenario. During her four-day ordeal, among the tortures that Margot endured were:

- a total of at least twenty hours of being whipped

- having both nipples pierced—several times each

- having her clitoris pierced

- having needles put under her fingernails

- being hung by her hair, with a 25-pound weight tied to her ankles

- having the entire front of her body slowly covered with hot wax

- having my initials branded into her flesh, one on the inside of each thigh

- being shocked repeatedly on her breasts and clitoris with an electric cattle prod.

I stayed with Margot an extra day longer than planned, giving myself two days to take care of her and make sure that she would be all right. On the night before I left, I very gently made love to her; afterward I told her that I very much wanted to keep on seeing her, but that I was also very worried about where she and I were heading. I told her that I wasn't sure that I would be able to keep my promise about doing anything to her that she asked, no matter how extreme.

Margot didn't give me any answer. Not then. Not ever. I never heard from her again. And two years later my Christmas card came back with "Not Deliverable" stamped on it.

I'm not sure, of course, but in my heart I think I know what happened to Margot. I think Margot is dead. I really believe that she found a new man with whom she found it possible to take her torture fantasies to their ultimate extreme.

In short, I think Margot found a man who recognized no limits whatever to the levels of brutality and sadism that he was willing to carry out and from whom Margot extracted the same promise that I had made her—that he would do to her whatever she asked.

And then I think one night he opened an envelope that read simply, "Torture me to death."

And he kept his promise.

12

Barbara

It's going to be very hard to write about Barbara.

It's going to be hard to make any sense out of the how and why and what of all the things that have happened between Barbara and me.

It's going to be hard to explain all the different Barbaras there have been during the last seventeen years.

Most of all, it's going to be hard to explain to people exactly how much I love her.

For openers I might explain that for eight years Barbara was my slave and that for the past nine years she's been my lover. But that hardly explains anything.

Inside, Barbara is the most beautiful person I have ever met. Outside, Barbara is very nice-looking, and when I met her she had about the sexiest body of any female I'd ever known.

Despite her good looks and the fact that she was then twenty-four years old, if I'd met Barbara two months earlier, I would have discovered that she was a virgin when she seduced me on our fourth date. She had only recently gotten up the nerve to move out of her home in Brooklyn and find her own tiny apartment in Manhattan. Shortly after that, deciding it was also time for her to find out what sex was all about, she had gone to bed with the bartender at the neighborhood saloon where she hung out after work.

I met Barbara in a coffee shop on Third Avenue. During our chat I learned that she worked for a New York radio station, that she was new to the city, and that she didn't have a steady boyfriend, so I called her two days later and invited her to dinner. She was very shy on that date and didn't talk much at first, but after a couple of drinks she relaxed enough so that I could coax some more history out of her.

Very simply, Barbara was an Irish Catholic girl from Brooklyn. She'd had a strict parochial school education and had been raised by old-fashioned Catholic parents who kept her very close to home. Her mother in particular had kept a very tight rein on her, and had colored Barbara's views of sex by explaining that intercourse was a thoroughly unpleasant and disgusting act which a woman engaged in only because it was one of the duties of a Catholic wife. As a result, Barbara had had very few dates and, until the bartender, her social contacts with men had pretty much been limited to a few movie dates and talking to the guys in her bowling league.

With that as a background, I should have realized that from Barbara's view I came across as a pretty scary type . . . a well-paid executive who had traveled all over the world and had done a lot of exciting things, who dressed well, drove a sporty car, ate in expensive restaurants, and had obviously had numerous exciting and exotic love affairs.

Of course, I didn't think of myself that way. If I had, I might have made a run at Barbara on that first date, but something about her told me to lay off. When we got back to her apartment, I shook her hand at the street door, said, "Thanks for a nice evening," kissed her lightly on the cheek, and walked away.

And that, according Barbara, is when she fell in love with me.

On our second date things were pretty much the same. A nice dinner, some pleasant talk, a slow walk home, and a goodnight kiss on the cheek at the street door. On the third date we went first to my apartment after dinner, where we sat on the couch for an hour or so and necked. It was then I discovered two things: first, Barbara had never kissed anyone with her mouth open. Second, from what I could tell without removing her blouse, she had the firmest, most beautifully shaped breasts of any woman I'd ever met. And this time, when I walked Barbara home, I took her upstairs to her apartment and kissed her goodnight there instead of at the street door.

On our fourth date Barbara seduced me. I had flown back to New

York at about 9:00 in the evening and had telephoned Barbara from La Guardia to see if she wanted to go out for a late cup of coffee. She said she'd rather stay home, but that I was welcome to stop by. When I got to her apartment at about ten o'clock, I was met by Barbara wearing the most incredibly sheer and sexy black lace "baby doll" pajamas.

I was right about her breasts!

We didn't get around to coffee until breakfast. This was the start of one of the most fascinating and exciting times of my life. I don't know whether I fully understood or appreciated this marvelous thing that had happened to me. It was the absolute fulfillment of every Master's wildest dream and fantasy. Here I was, a 34-year-old man with a lovely new 24-year-old girlfriend who was totally in love with me. She was completely inexperienced in every area of sensual activity, and utterly willing and eager to learn and experience absolutely anything I wanted her to learn for my pleasure.

Barbara had slept with only one man before she met me, and she had been with him only half a dozen times at most. She had never had an orgasm; even more incredible, she'd never even masturbated. But after two months, she was having multiple orgasms regularly, screaming her joy and pleasure with total abandon. (To this day Barbara puts her hand over her mouth when my cock first enters her to smother the cry she always makes.)

Barbara had always been embarrassed by her beautiful body, but after three months she was wearing the most provocative outfits, loving the attention it brought her and the pleasure it brought me. It was the year of the see-through blouse, which was made for women like Barbara. She was five feet three inches tall with a slender 105-pound body. But my God, her breasts! Full and high and beautifully shaped, and so incredibly firm that despite the fact that she more than filled a 34B cup, she looked absolutely no different without a bra. When Barbara walked into a cocktail party wearing the smoky, sheer, see-through blouse I had picked out for her, every man in the room got a hard-on and every woman in the room got a headache.

Barbara had never even French-kissed a man, but after four months she was more talented at oral sex than anyone I've ever met before or since. Linda Lovelace hadn't come along yet, so Barbara had to invent the "deep throat" technique all by herself. I remember telling other men about it, but no one believed me until the movie was released years later.

Barbara had never heard of bondage, but after five months I was tying her to my bed on occasion before making love to her. I learned how to bring her to the very peak of an orgasm and then hold her there, sometimes for as long as ten minutes or more. At other times I would bring her to as many fifteen or twenty completely separate orgasms in the space of less than one hour!

And, of course, Barbara had never even dreamed of anything like "S/M," but after six months she was hanging by her wrists from the rings in the ceiling of my apartment, her naked body drenched in sweat and almost entirely covered by the marks of my cat-o'-nine-tails.

I admit it. Our relationship was totally one-sided. Barbara literally worshiped the ground I stood on and she devoted every minute of her life to serving my pleasure. I loved her, but she loved me so much more! Never in my life have I ever been so totally and obviously adored, and I just plain took advantage of it.

Although I had no other slaves at the time, I was dating some other "straight" girls, and more than once I'd have a date with one of them, make love, and then leave and show up at Barbara's in the middle of the night. I was never questioned. I was simply welcomed into her apartment and into her arms and into her bed and into her body. The next morning she opened a beer for herself and poured me a glass of orange juice, and then she gently sucked my cock while I sipped the juice and lay there feeling all big and powerful and wonderful.

Shit, it got so I really believed I deserved it!

I repeat . . . I honestly loved Barbara. In private it wasn't all whips and domination. I helped her find a new and better job when she was suddenly fired by the radio station. I introduced her to things she'd never been exposed to . . . the theater and opera and books. And in public I went out of my way to make sure everyone knew that she was my girl and how proud I was of her. For the first time in her life Barbara felt loved and adored, and she bloomed!

But still it was mostly a one-way street, and I took total advantage of the power I had over this selfless and loving lady. Once, early on in our relationship, I accidentally found out she'd made a dinner date with a girl in her office. I deliberately waited until five minutes to five that afternoon before calling Barbara and telling her I wanted her to be in my apartment at six o'clock. When she asked why, I said, "Because I feel like whipping someone." "But I have a date," she said. "Break it," I told her, and hung up.

When Barbara showed up at ten minutes before six, I tied her up with her arms over her head, and so taut that her toes were just touching the floor. Then I left her hanging there for nearly an hour while I went out for a cheeseburger and a couple of beers. When I came back, I whipped her before taking her down and taking her to bed.

It was a perfect dominant/submissive relationship, except maybe for the fact that Barbara drank a lot. But then, so did I, and it produced some wild times. For instance, one night we were invited to a huge party at the old Dom in lower Manhattan. It was thrown by some high-fashion dress manufacturing company and a number of the female guests were models who were wearing a wide variety of fairly revealing outfits . . . dresses slit to the navel, see-through blouses, and the like. The trouble is that many high-fashion models don't have that much to reveal.

However, it was fun, and all went well until Barbara and I tried to start a polite conversation with a group of models and their dates, only to be totally and obviously snubbed. Apparently we weren't their type, and they pointedly let us know it. At that point, Barbara, who had had several drinks, took me aside and asked me for twenty dollars. When I asked her what for, she said, "You'll see, but I want to run home. You guard the door to make sure I can get back in and I'll be back as soon as I can."

I camped out downstairs by the door. Nearly an hour later Barbara came back, grinning from ear to ear. "What the hell did you do?" I asked. "Check this," she answered, and she yanked open her raincoat like a flasher. From the waist down she was wearing black bikini panties over a pair of black full-length open lace tights. Above the waist she was wearing a half a dozen gold chains of various lengths. Other than that, she was naked.

Except for one thing. She had carefully accented her nipples with lipstick in order to make her breasts even more startlingly beautiful . . . and noticeable.

"Holy shit!" I finally said.

Barbara grinned again and casually tossed her raincoat to the hatcheck lady. "Come on," she said. "Le's go show those flat-chested fuckers what a *real* woman is supposed to look like." And up the stairs she went, with me, still in shock, following her.

By then the band was in full swing. All the pretty people were doing the frug or whatever the "in" dance was back then, and we joined them. Holding a tumbler half full of straight Scotch that she'd picked up at the bar, Barbara went out on the dance floor, deliberately picked one of the daringly dressed models who had snubbed us earlier, and then just danced next to her, sipping at her drink with a totally innocent expression on her face while those magnificent breasts drew all the admiring attention that had, until then, been focused on the other girl. The model promptly decided she'd danced enough and left the floor while Barbara picked out another target.

On average, it took about two minutes for each "victim" to figure it out and leave the floor. A couple of them tried to move away while still dancing, but Barbara simply moved with them. In less than half an hour, six or eight snooty models had been driven to cover. Barbara and I were surrounded by two dozen admiring men who, when the music finally stopped, spontaneously broke into applause while Barbara grinned, chug-a-lugged the last two ounces of her Scotch, and strutted off the dance floor.

Just about then two things happened. First, one of the hosts took me aside and told me he thought maybe Barbara had gone a little too far. Second, almost simultaneously, the drinks caught up to Barbara, who just made it to the ladies room before throwing up.

So we left. Barbara had made herself sick a couple of times before by drinking too much, and on those occasions I'd whipped her severely as punishment. But this time she'd been so much fun that I just couldn't do it. And the next morning, Barbara was fine . . . wandering around the apartment sipping on her customary morning beer and humming along to the radio.

My domination of Barbara grew in intensity. Once I ordered her to write a note detailing some activity designed to please me and bring it to me at my apartment. Here's what she wrote:

Dear John,

I want you to stand me on a chair and tie my wrists to the rings in the ceiling. Then I want you to tie my ankles together so that I can't kick. Then blindfold me. Then I want you to pull the chair away so that I'm hanging by my wrists, and then I want you to whip me as hard as you want and as long as you want. I want you to whip my bottom and whip my back and whip my legs and whip my belly and whip my breasts. And if I scream I want you to gag me, and if I

faint I want you to wait for me to come to and then keep on whipping
me, and I don't want you to stop as long as you are having fun. I
love you.

Barbara

That note was hardly inventive. It simply asked me to do exactly what
I'd done many times before, with a frequency that resulted in there
always being at least one bruise or welt on Barbara's body put there
by me.

I loved disciplining Barbara, but all the signs pointed to it being
as exciting for her as it was for me. All I had to do was tie her up
and the juices would start flowing in her pussy. Sometimes she would
actually have an orgasm while I was whipping her and she told me
that whenever she masturbated, she would fantasize about me tying
her up and whipping her.

But I kept constantly raising the ante, slowly increasing the intensity and severity of the discipline, almost as if I were trying to see how
far I could go before Barbara would leave me. I'd read the *Story of
O*, of course, so when I was feeling particularly sadistic I'd tie Barbara with her legs spread apart and whip the inside of her thighs. Later
I read *The Image,* and I promptly began torturing Barbara by using
heated needles on her breasts and nipples. But Barbara never broke;
and each time, when I had finally stopped the torture, Barbara would
kneel before me and hug my legs, telling me how much she loved me.

Eventually, of course, I gave Barbara to others to whip, enjoying
the kick of demonstrating my total power over her. The only thing I
didn't do was give her to others to use sexually. Somewhere along the
line I'd promised Barbara that I wouldn't let any other man or woman
make love to her, and I never broke that promise. But every couple
of months or so would find Barbara hanging by her wrists, naked, blindfolded, and gagged, while as many as four men took turns whipping
her. Once I took her to dinner with three other men. After our order
had been taken, I explained to Barbara that after dinner all of us were
going to whip her. Barbara had been ordered not to talk, and so for
the next two hours the other three men and I casually discussed what
we were planning to do to her . . . how she would be tied and how
she would be tormented. We talked among ourselves as if Barbara weren't
even there, while she just sat and listened. After dinner we took her
back to the apartment and played with her exactly as we had planned.

Barbara changed jobs three more times. Between jobs she'd work as a temporary, and during those periods she accompanied me on my business trips: Miami, Atlanta, Los Angeles, Houston, Nassau, Chicago, New Orleans, Providence, Fort Lauderdale, Philadelphia, Montreal, Boston, San Francisco, Dallas, and Mexico City. I took my wonderful slave to all these places. In each city she was whipped. In each city I was worshiped.

We celebrated Barbara's thirtieth birthday on a Friday night in New Orleans. We'd been there together several times before, and it was a special place for us. We had cocktails at the lovely Royal Orleans Hotel and dinner at Antoine's. After dinner we strolled Bourbon Street for a couple of hours listening to jazz before going back to our suite at the old Bourbon Orleans Hotel.

At dinner Barbara told me that she had a "reverse birthday present" for me, but that the present was at the hotel because she wanted to wait to give it to me until the end of the evening. Shortly after we returned to the hotel, Barbara went upstairs to the bedroom. When she returned she was naked and was carrying a very thin, flexible bamboo rod. She knelt in front of me and explained that while everyone should of course be spanked on their birthday, slaves should properly be spanked in a very special way. Consequently, she had gone to the Pleasure Chest and selected this cane, hoping that I would enjoy using it on her ass a total of thirty-one times . . . one for each year since her birth plus one to grow on. I told her I'd be delighted.

Barbara pulled the large stuffed armchair into the middle of the living room and knelt facing it, wrapping her arms around the back. She turned her head to look at me, smiled, and whispered, "Happy birthday, love"; and then she buried her head in the seat of the chair waiting for the first stroke.

As soon as the bamboo switch cut into her ass the first time, we both knew Barbara had made a mistake. She later told me that the pain was worse than anything she had ever experienced. I was used to Barbara handling even the most severe discipline with a fair degree of stoicism, but when the cane landed her whole body jumped and a scream was literally torn out of her. I waited maybe ten seconds before delivering the second stroke, and this time, although her body jumped again, Barbara managed not to cry out. She also remained quiet for the third and fourth strokes. But when the fifth one landed she jerked so violently that the whole chair moved, her head came up, and she screamed and cried out, "Oh, God! Oh, God!" several times. Tears were running down her cheeks and her whole body was trembling. "Do you want me to stop?" I asked her.

Barbara continued to cry. "I can't take back your present but I don't think I'm going to be able to handle it, either," she told me through her tears. Hugging the chair, she buried her face in the seat again.

I hit her the sixth and seventh time, spacing the strokes out to give her body a chance to adjust to the pain, but each time she screamed. On the eighth stroke she let go of the back of the chair and, while still kneeling, straightened her upper body and held her arms in front of her. Her fists were clenched and she was trembling all over, shaking her head slowly back and forth. Her eyes were closed, her mouth was open, and her face was covered with tears as I heard her whispering, "Please, please, please, please, please."

"Please, what?" I asked her. She continued to cry, and finally she lowered her head into the seat of the chair again. "Please, what?" I asked again.

"Oh, God, I don't know," she said.

"Just ask me to stop," I told her.

Barbara shook her head. "Oh, God, I can't, I can't," she said, still crying. "I can't take back your present."

I bound and gagged her. I strapped her knees tightly to the front legs of the chair and tied her arms around the back. Then I strapped the gag in place and put an extra pillow under her head.

I used the cane on her ass twenty-three more times. Even though I tried to hold back, it was agony for her. I moved the switch from place to place, trying not to cut her twice in the same spot; some of the strokes landed on her upper thighs, but those hurt her even more. I took my time, giving Barbara a chance to recover from each stroke and get ready for the next one, but it didn't really help that much. I wanted to stop but I also knew that I had to finish. However, unlike most of the times I've disciplined a woman, this wasn't much fun.

After the thirtieth stroke I waited a long time, and then I delivered the last one, and I was almost glad when Barbara fainted. At least it ended her pain for a while.

Her ass looked horrible . . . the worst I'd ever seen. There was no blood, but the skin was broken in several places and her entire bottom was covered with ugly red welts that were already beginning to turn purple. While Barbara was still tied and unconscious, I got a warm washcloth and some soap, and I gently washed her and then put some of my shaving lotion on to try to prevent an infection. As I did it, I was glad she was still out because I knew that if she'd been conscious, the pain of the alcohol in the lotion would have been unbearable.

I untied her, carried her upstairs, and laid her gently face down on the bed. I sat next to her and gently stroked her head and her back while waiting for her to come to.

She did, finally, after maybe five minutes, and when she first tried to roll over I put my hands on her shoulders and held her still, telling her not to move. She turned her head and looked at me. "God, I hurt," she whispered.

"I know," I said.

"How bad is it?" she asked.

"Pretty bad," I told her. "The worst I've ever seen."

Barbara thought about that for a while, and then she reached out and took my hand. "Tell me something," she whispered. "If I'd asked you to, would you have stopped?"

"Yes."

"I thought so," she said, and then she almost smiled as she added, "You're not so tough."

"I'm a pussycat," I told her. She squeezed my hand and then pulled it to her lips and kissed it. Then she looked at me. "Do me a favor?" she asked."

"Anything."

"Get me a very big and very stiff drink."

Barbara was drunk by the time she went to sleep, but she still cried out several times during the night. After we got back to New York, it was four days before she could go back to work.

It finally occurred to me that Barbara's drinking was far beyond the ordinary. One morning, I accidentally picked up her orange juice instead of mine and discovered it was half vodka. This explained why she'd given up her morning can of beer. That spring, Barbara had gotten sick and been in the hospital a couple of days, and in the fall she went in again. This time the doctor told me flat out that Barbara was an alcoholic and that she needed help.

I tried very hard to get her to cut down on her drinking. It didn't work, but finally I did convince her to go to a psychiatrist who, in turn, referred her to Alcoholics Anonymous. I figured that was going to solve things.

I was so wrong!

First, it seems Barbara was scared to death of AA and had to get drunk before she could go to the meetings. But much, much worse was that her psychiatrist didn't understand alcoholism: his answer to her drinking was to put her on tranquilizers. So, toward the end, although I didn't know it at the time, Barbara was taking eight to ten pills a day and also going through as much as a quart and a half of vodka. She is very lucky to be alive!

It was an awful period. Barbara was drunk most of the time and the only way I could be sure of her getting to the doctor or to AA meetings was to take her myself. It was a fight all the way, and more than once Barbara would try to convince me that it would be more fun if I'd just take her home and whip her. But I had stopped doing that; I'd also pretty much stopped making love to her. Since she was no longer having orgasms, it wasn't any fun for me any more.

Worst of all, I was absolutely convinced that I was entirely to blame for Barbara's alcoholism. In short, I'd taken this beautiful, sensitive, generous, loving girl and, by turning her into my slave, I'd also turned her into a drunk.

The bottom came the next spring. When I called Barbara at her temporary job, I was advised, rather testily, that she was lying unconscious on the floor under her desk; if I was someone responsible for her, they'd appreciate my doing something about it. I called Barbara's AA sponsor, and together we arranged to get her into a hospital. Next, her sponsor arranged to have Barbara admitted to an alcoholic treatment center in Connecticut. Five days later, I checked Barbara out of the hospital in New York and drove her to the center. I stayed with her while they admitted her, and then I kissed her goodbye and left.

Barbara stayed there five weeks. On Wednesday of the last week, she called me to tell me she'd be taking the train back to New York that Saturday, and to ask if I could meet her at Grand Central Station.

I'll never forget it! I'd gotten used to Barbara walking in the manner so typical of alcoholics . . . her shoulders hunched and her head down, looking as if she expected someone to hit her at any moment. But here came Barbara, striding across that huge Grand Central waiting area, her shoulders back, her head up, her suitcase slung over her shoulder, and a huge grin on her face. God, did she look marvelous!

We went directly to my apartment and fucked for three hours, and then we went to her apartment and fucked the rest of the night. On

Sunday I tied her up and whipped her gently all afternoon. She had five orgasms while I was whipping her and two more afterward while I made love to her. It was all back together and it was wonderful!

The next few weeks were like a second honeymoon. I saw Barbara almost every day and stayed with her two or three nights each week. Every minute we spent together was so highly charged that you could almost taste it.

The sex was incredible and the "S/M" even more intense than before. To celebrate our "new beginning" I bought Barbara a silver slave collar. The night I gave it to her, I stood her on a footstool with both wrists tied together and chained to one of the ceiling rings. Every few minutes I'd take away the footstool to leave Barbara completely suspended, and then I'd push her body to make it slowly turn. Her head was thrown back, her breasts were pulled high, and her belly muscles were stretched taut by the weight of her suspended body.

A single candle was burning on the coffee table and its light reflected from the perspiration that covered Barbara's naked flesh as she slowly twisted there at the end of the chain. Each time her body turned to face me I'd bring the whip down across her breasts or belly.

I'd whip her that way for two or three minutes, and then I'd put the footstool back and let her stand on it while I used my fingers in her ass and her cunt, frequently bringing her to still another orgasm before I pulled the stool away and picked up the whip again. It went on that way for almost four hours, and during that entire time, whether I was whipping her or making love to her, all Barbara ever said was, "Oh, God, I love it! I love it! I love it!" over and over and over again.

It was the best ever!

Four months after Barbara's homecoming, we went to Acapulco for a long weekend. On the way down, Barbara asked if I could possibly manage not to whip her until the last night, and I agreed. That last night I chose to whip her in a way that had always been very special for both of us. I had her make love to me a while by sucking my cock until it was fully erect, and then I had her take top and handcuffed her hands behind her. Then I used a small whip on her breasts and belly while she "rode" me.

I loved doing it that way. I'd lie there looking up at Barbara with those beautiful breasts arched outward by her bound arms. She'd lean her head back and I'd feel the strength and tension in her thighs as

they worked to slowly raise and lower her body on my cock. Each
time the whip hit her, she'd smile and grind her hips against mine before
raising her body again.

I've always had pretty good control in that position and with Barbara I could sometimes keep it up for an hour or more, during which
time the entire front of Barbara's upper body would slowly become
covered with welts while she experienced an almost continuous stream
of orgasms. This was one of those special times, and it went on and
on. After about half an hour, I stopped the whipping and started using
needles to carefully torment her nipples. Barbara began a steady low
moan that was produced by that lovely combination of the pain of
the needles in her breasts and the pleasure of my cock in her pussy.

Barbara had two tremendous orgasms, with her body's response
to the second one actually tumbling her off me, but I pulled her back
onto me and picked up the whip to start again. That's when Barbara
began to cry and, for the first time ever, I heard her begging me not
to whip her any more.

What I didn't realize right away was that Barbara didn't just want
me to stop whipping her that night. She wanted me to stop whipping
her *forever*.

We talked the rest of the night and most of the next day. Very
simply, Barbara was afraid that if she continued to be my "slave," she'd
start drinking again. She explained that most alcoholics have a very
low image of themselves, which contributes to their drinking problem.
She was quick to add that she had never felt demeaned by being my
slave. Instead, it had always been a tremendous source of pride and
pleasure for her. But despite that, she had, over the last four months,
realized that the submission, the whipping, and the drinking were
somehow all very closely tied together. Barbara told me she was afraid
that if she kept it up she would start drinking again, and that if she
did she would die.

That was the bottom line.

We stayed in Acapulco an extra day. Barbara cried most of the
time and, finally, she told me she was terribly afraid that if she stopped
being my slave, I'd leave her. She said she knew how important being
her Master was to me, and she didn't see how I could ever have her
any other way.

I answered her in the only way I knew. I put the two whips, the
pair of handcuffs, her slave collar, and the needles in a pillowcase and

tied a knot in the top. Then I pulled on a pair of slacks, told Barbara to put on her dungarees and a T-shirt, grabbed a blanket, and together we went for a walk on the beach. North of the hotel where we were staying is a long stretch of beach. I took Barbara's hand as we slowly walked barefoot along the edge of the ocean until we reached a place where we were all alone. It was about eight o'clock at night, the ocean was calm with only tiny waves, and an almost full moon rose low in the sky to the south out over the water.

Kissing Barbara lightly, I waded into the water and swung the pillowcase around my head three or four times before throwing it as far out into the ocean as I could. Then I led Barbara to a little valley between two sand dunes where I spread the blanket out. Slowly stripping Barbara, I laid her down on the blanket and then I took off my own clothes. I was already very erect. I slowly knelt between Barbara's legs, kissed her mouth and both breasts, and then, very gently and very slowly, I made love to her.

Afterward, lying on top of her with my softened cock still inside her, I took Barbara's face in my hands and kissed her one more time. And then I said, "I love you, Barbara, and from now on you are my lover, not my slave, and we will never talk about it again."

For nine years I've kept my word. Barbara is still my lover and I hope she always will be, because she is more special and precious to me than I can possibly tell her.

Best of all, Barbara is still sober. She has never touched a drink and in a few months it will be ten years.

And when Barbara reads this, she'll remind me for the thousandth time that talking about the future is the wrong way to think. It is only today that counts.

13

Vanessa and Patty

I took Vanessa to New Orleans for a long S/M weekend. To make sure that our time in the Crescent City was doubly entertaining, I arranged to take along an extra "slave," Patty H____, whose regular Master/husband, Jim, owed me several favors and who, even without such obligations, took tremendous pleasure from "dispatching" his slave/wife to serve other trusted dominants. Vanessa was in rare form. She knew, of course, that she would be expected to serve my pleasure in various ways, but she also knew that she would have her own "servant." I had made it clear to Vanessa that she would be given the right to dominate Patty totally in any way she chose, and that Patty would be the prime target of discipline activities for the weekend. In effect, Vanessa and I were going as two fellow dominants, taking our slave with us. So Vanessa was on a high, and from the very beginning she played her part. Patty carried Vanessa's bags from the taxi, walking behind her. Patty accompanied Vanessa to the ladies room and "attended" her there. Patty fetched Vanessa a drink at the airport. And in a fine symbolic gesture, Vanessa had arranged for herself and me to fly first class while Patty rode in the tourist section.

But there was a hitch. Just before the trip I'd had some rather serious personal problems; so while Vanessa was having a ball, I was feeling quite down, which, of course, was no way to start that kind of an adventure. Vanessa sensed my mood immediately and determined to do something about it. She tried jokes. She tried booze. She tried sexy conversation. Nothing was working. But about half an hour before landing, she came up with a different kind of an idea.

"How would you like to see Patty whip me?" she suddenly asked. It was something that had never occurred to me, and it caught me off guard.

"Patty whip you?" I asked.

"Yeah," Vanessa answered. "Hell, John, you're on a downer and if you don't snap out of it, you're going to fuck up the whole weekend. So I have an idea that I think will be a lot of fun for you."

"Patty whipping you?" I asked again.

"Yes. You know damn well just the idea alone turns you on," Vanessa said, "but it's more than that. Look, what I thought was that tonight you could make up some excuse about something I'd done to make you angry and that you were changing the rules. Instead of me automatically being the boss, you'd arrange a contest between Patty and me to see who got to be the slave for the weekend."

I was beginning to be interested. "Go on," I told her.

"See, it's working already," Vanessa laughed. "The way I figure it, you'd give her an hour to dominate me and then I'd have an hour to dominate her. Then you could decide who had done the best job."

"What if you lose?" I asked.

"I fucking well better not, you asshole!" Vanessa said, "or I'll never speak to you again."

I thought about it for a while. Vanessa was right. The prospect was definitely improving my mood. Then, just before the plane landed, Vanessa made an interesting change in the plot. "Hey, John," she said, "I've got an even better idea."

"What's that?"

"Let me whip Patty first."

"Why?"

"So she'll have a reason to get even," Vanessa explained. "I'm going to kick the shit out of her so I know that she'll be hard on me, and that way it will be the most fun for you." As I've said before, Vanessa was a dead game lady.

That's the way we played it. I'd reserved a lovely duplex suite at the Bourbon Orleans Hotel, with two-story high French doors leading out to a second-story balcony overlooking Bourbon Street and a staircase leading up to the king-sized bed on the second deck. After we'd unpacked, I called the girls together and announced the contest. But instead of automatically letting Vanessa go first, I decided to let "chance" decide. The old phony coin flip again, and of course Vanessa was chosen to have first crack at Patty.

After ordering Patty to strip, Vanessa then asked me to help tie her. At Vanessa's request we stood Patty next to the stairs and used the open railing on the balcony to tie her arms over her head. We had no place to tie Patty's ankles so Vanessa simply tied them together. Finally, I allowed Vanessa to use a blindfold but I vetoed the gag. After all, how was I going to judge fairly?

True to her word, Vanessa did, indeed, "kick the shit out of Patty." She used the riding crop exclusively over and over again until Patty was covered front and back with thin red stripes. Occasionally she'd take a brief rest and ask Patty if she wanted to quit, thereby giving up her chance at Vanessa. I think that Patty might have quit, except that she was more afraid of what I'd do to her if she did, so she hung in. At the end, Patty was screaming, and so at last I did allow Vanessa to use the gag.

I was more than a little interested to see what Patty would do to Vanessa. I'd never seen Patty take the dominant role, but I'd heard that she enjoyed it, and I was frankly looking forward to it. Before the two traded roles, however, I called a timeout, ordered them both to take showers, and then took them both up to the bedroom and had them take turns going down on me until I came, finally, in Patty's mouth.

It was time now for the second inning. Vanessa had deliberately set herself up for a heavy session and she was ready to take her medicine. "Remember, John, this one's for you," Vanessa whispered to me on her way back down the stairs. "I hope you enjoy it."

"Oh, I will," I assured her. "More than you know."

She didn't understand what I meant until after she had been tied in exactly the same way Patty had been tied. Then I added the kicker: "Patty," I said, "you have one hour to make Vanessa say 'please.' If you don't, I'm going to give you to her for the rest of the weekend."

I heard Vanessa suck in her breath. "You son of a bitch!" she murmured.

"Go to it, Patty," I said in response, smiling at Vanessa.

Patty went to it, using the same riding crop at first, and then changing to a cat, and finally to a short dog whip that I knew hurt terribly and which Patty used on Vanessa's breasts until I stopped her. As "referee," I had the right to step in, but Vanessa still took a hell of a beating. With fifteen minutes left, Patty had a new idea, and with my help we stood Vanessa on a chair and shortened the ropes holding her arms to the upper railing. Then Patty pulled the chair away, leaving Vanessa hanging by her wrists, her feet about a foot off the floor, and she picked up the cat again.

That's when I decided to go out on the balcony, and what followed provided me with one of the most erotic memories I have of all my S/M experiences. The huge French doors had full-length sheer curtains and there was a light behind the two girls. It was impossible to see them in detail, but the two silhouettes were very clear—the outline of Vanessa's extended body, hanging by the wrists, her head thrown back with her long hair almost touching her waist, and the shadowy form of Patty as she slowly walked around the helpless body of her victim, swinging the whip over and over again into Vanessa's naked flesh.

Vanessa won, of course. At the end she, too, was screaming, but I denied her the gag and she never said "please." I had them shower again and go down on me once more. Then the three of us went across Bourbon Street to a bar called Lucky Pierre's for Irish coffee and some piano music. Both Patty and Vanessa wore see-through blouses that showed the welts criss-crossing their bodies if you looked closely, as several people did. We were definitely the talk of the piano bar.

Back at the hotel I finally "presented" Patty to Vanessa, who thanked me and then ordered Patty to strip, kneel before her, and kiss both her feet. "Now for the finale," Vanessa said. She had already decided on her plans for the remainder of the evening. They were really very simple. With my help we stood Patty on the same chair and tied her arms to the balcony railing just as Vanessa had been tied, except that at Vanessa's request we used towels to pad Patty's wrists. I soon found out why.

Once Patty was ready, Vanessa asked me to go upstairs and get ready for bed. I did as she asked. When I came out of the bathroom and looked down from the balcony into the living room, nothing had changed. Patty was still standing on the chair and Vanessa was relaxing on the couch. "I'm ready," I called down.

"Fine," said Vanessa. She got up and walked over to Patty. "Goodnight, slave," she said, and she pulled away the chair, leaving Patty swinging by her wrists. Then she turned off the living room lights and came upstairs.

"How long are you going to leave her hanging there?" I asked Vanessa.

She grinned at me. "Until I've finished making love to you," she said.

"How long do you figure that will be?"

"Well," Vanessa said with a chuckle, "you've already come twice tonight and you had three Drambuies at Pierre's. So if I take it slow, I figure you might last all night."

Actually I lasted for more than an hour, and for that entire time Patty hung down there in the living room. She never made a sound. After my orgasm, Vanessa went down, untied Patty, and ordered her to go to the bathroom. While Patty was gone, Vanessa converted the living room couch into a bed and when Patty came back, Vanessa used a pair of handcuffs to fasten one of Patty's wrists to the frame. Then she tucked Patty in, kissed her goodnight, and came back upstairs.

"I'm surprised Patty didn't make any noise hanging there that long," I told Vanessa after we were in bed.

"I'm not," Vanessa answered.

"How come?"

Vanessa snuggled up close to me. "Because I told her if she made one fucking sound I'd come down and brand her nipples with a cigarette." I don't know if Vanessa would actually have done that, but obviously Patty had been convinced that she would.

Since I had arranged a golf match the next day with a friend in New Orleans, I was gone all day. I left Vanessa and Patty together, and they had a fine time as I heard later . . . breakfast at Brennan's, a ride on a Mississippi paddle wheeler, and shopping along Canal Street. All of the time, of course, Vanessa was the lady and Patty was her servant.

Dinner that night was in a small private dining room at Antoine's, where Vanessa continued playing her role to the hilt. Vanessa had ordered Patty to come to dinner wearing only a blouse and skirt with no underwear, and while Vanessa and I were eating Oysters Rockefeller, Patty was on her knees eating Vanessa.

She went down on me for dessert.

We returned to Pierre's for after-dinner drinks and some singing. Finally, at about eleven o'clock, we went back to the hotel, where Va-

nessa began her feature act. She had spent the entire day preparing
for the evening and doing a psych job on Patty to ensure her coopera-
tion. Vanessa asked me to sit next to her on the couch while Patty
got herself ready. It didn't really take much. Patty simply went upstairs, took a quick shower, and then came back down, still naked,
and knelt in front of us. "Please, Master John," she said, "I would
like to beg your permission to have Mistress Vanessa torture me for
the rest of the night."

I gave my consent.

It was the first time I'd ever seen Vanessa really let loose on another woman. I'd often seen her reduce a male submissive to tears and
screams; but usually that was simply the result of a long and brutal
flogging with her riding crop, carried out until the male subject "broke."
With Patty it was much more involved. She started by strapping Patty
to the top of the living room table, her legs pulled wide to expose
her pussy. Next she took the vibrator that Patty had brought with her
and used it on Patty's clit until Patty had her first orgasm, at which
point Vanessa asked me to take the vibrator and keep Patty coming
while she began the "torture." Patty was one of those women who have
orgasms very easily, and she was also able to have almost endless multiple orgasms, one coming right on top of the other. That was the state
Patty was in when I took over the vibrator and Vanessa went to work.

That afternoon Vanessa had read to Patty the section of the book
The Image, where Anne has her breasts tortured by Claire using needles.
Vanessa had told Patty that she planned to torture her breasts and
nipples in the same way, and she had ordered Patty to go to the store
and buy some needles for her. Patty obediently returned from the 5-
and-10 with two large packs, each containing nearly one hundred needles
of every conceivable size. And so, while I used the vibrator to keep
Patty in what amounted to a constant orgasm, Vanessa began tormenting Patty's nipples by pricking them repeatedly with the sharpest needles.
Patty soon began a steady shrill whine, but it seemed more related
to the sensations in her pussy than the torment of her nipples.

Finally, Vanessa began actually putting needles into Patty's nipples
and breasts, dipping the points first in alcohol and then inserting them
into Patty's flesh, embedding each one perhaps one-eighth or one-quar-
ter of an inch deep. That's when Patty began fighting the straps that
held her to the table and the whine became punctuated with screams
each time her breast was pierced. Vanessa asked me to gag Patty and

after I did, she continued. Half an hour or so later, there were perhaps twenty-five needles in each of Patty's breasts, a few in each of the two aureoles around Patty's nipples but most of them in the breasts themselves, which looked now like very sensuous pin cushions.

"I don't think there's room for any more," Vanessa said at last, studying the results of her efforts, "but there's one more thing I've always wanted to do to a girl and now's my chance."

"What's that?" I asked.

"Actually pierce her nipples . . . put a needle all the way through them. And by God, I'm going to do it!"

Vanessa proceeded to remove all the needles from Patty's breasts and then she washed them both with alcohol. Finally she took a long, slightly heavier needle and, holding Patty's left nipple between her thumb and forefinger, began trying to pass the needle completely through the base of the nipple itself. Patty was obviously in agony, screaming into the gag and fighting desperately against the straps that were holding her almost motionless to the table top. What was fascinating to me was that at the same time, Patty was still apparently continuing her endless string of orgasms caused by the vibrator that I was still using on her clitoris. I could see the muscles of her lower belly clenching and unclenching in a steady rhythm that had nothing to do with her effort to escape the torture that was being inflicted on her upper body.

It took a very long time. I don't think either of us had any idea how terribly hard it would be, but despite using a very sharp needle it took several minutes and every bit of Vanessa's strength to force the needle through what was obviously the very tough flesh of Patty's nipple. Actually, Vanessa was able to do it only by using a cork to brace one side of the nipple and a thimble from her sewing kit to help her push the needle through.

I think both Vanessa and I were relieved when it was finally done, and no way was either of us ready to pierce Patty's other nipple. As a matter of fact, I learned later that Vanessa had made several other plans for Patty that evening; but after piercing that one nipple, there was sort of an unspoken agreement between us that enough was enough. So the needle was removed as gently as possible, Patty's breasts were again carefully cleaned with a disinfectant, and she was untied.

The evening ended with all of us taking showers and then going to bed together in the king-size bed. Usually when I'm in bed with two women I take the middle, but this time Vanessa and I put Patty between us and we both made love to her. Together we kissed and gently stroked Patty's entire body. Then Vanessa went down on her while I carefully made love to those same breasts that Vanessa had tortured so severely earlier. After Vanessa's tongue had brought Patty to several more orgasms, we traded and I took top and very gently fucked Patty while Vanessa used her soft long hair and her tongue alternately to caress Patty's face and breasts and body. Considering what we had done to Patty earlier that evening, I know it sounds strange, but it was really very good, warm, gentle, and loving for all of us.

And what I remember most about that last part of the evening was just before we went to sleep when Patty, with total sincerity, hugged and kissed both Vanessa and me in turn and then said, "Thank you, Mistress Vanessa. Thank you, Master John. Thank you both for bringing me to New Orleans. I've had a lovely time."

14

Marsha

Several years ago, I moved to Chicago. I kept the apartment in SoHo but I also established a similar apartment in Chicago's "Near North" section. Shortly thereafter, I met Marsha and shared an affair with her for almost a year.

We accidentally met again three years later, and I mentioned to her that I was writing this book. A couple of weeks after our meeting, Marsha telephoned me at my office and told me that she had kept a "journal" ever since she was in junior high school, and that she thought her written record of our times together might be of interest.

She was right.

Jan. 9

I had lunch with a new man today. His name is John Q____ and I met him in the Pump Room the week before Christmas when Patty and I met there for drinks. He's older than me, about forty-five, and not spectacular looking. But he has incredibly beautiful green eyes and some gray in his hair that might make him look rather distinguished if he dressed better. But there's something about him. I'm not sure what. Maybe it's just that he seems so confident of himself and that's always a turn-on. At any rate, he's married, too, so at least if something comes of it we'll both be on equal ground. But I doubt that anything will.

Jan. 17

Dinner with John Q. Cocktails at the Pump Room and then over to Sage's restaurant. God, can he talk! But fascinating! He's been in advertising all his life and he tells the most marvelously funny stories. And something else. Unlike all the other married men I've ever dated, he told me flat out that he loves his wife. It's like me with Harry. I love Harry but sometimes I just get a terrible itch for something different. But I don't know about John that way. First, he's almost twenty years older than me. And second, he shook my hand goodnight! I wonder if he's a secret gay?

Jan. 30

Dinner with John again. This time at Hy's and we sat at the piano bar afterward and talked forever! I really think I like him, and I think he likes me. But another goddamn handshake at the garage! Maybe the asshole doesn't realize that I am one of the best damn looking 30-year-old women in Chicago. But he did touch me now and then, and he has the strongest hands I've ever felt. I wonder if I'm headed for trouble again?

Feb. 12

John again! I think the son of a bitch has got me hooked! We had a dinner date, and at eleven o'clock this morning a messenger showed up in my office with a single yellow rose and a card that said, "Thanks for making tonight special." We had dinner up at the Clark Street Cafe, and during dinner John told me for the first time that he had an in-town apartment and that it was only a couple of blocks away. Then came the zinger! I asked him if he was going to show me his apartment and he said, "Not tonight," and when I asked why he said, "Because tonight you are so beautiful and I want you so much that I wouldn't let you leave and you'd get in trouble with Harry." But this time he kissed me goodnight. God, did he kiss me goodnight.! He's strong as a bull and I leaked all over the fucking car seat all the way home. So much for his being gay! When Harry got home, I practically raped him. The poor dear never knew what hit him!

Feb. 19

John called me at work just before quitting time and asked me to go out the night after next. When I asked him where we would be going he said, "To my apartment. I think it's time we went to bed." And then the bastard hung up. Fuck him!

Feb. 20

I'm such an asshole! I called John first thing this morning and told him that I wasn't going out with him tomorrow. He said OK. Then I called him just before lunch and told him that I would go out but that I didn't want to go to his apartment. He said OK. Then I called him after lunch and said that we could go to his apartment but that didn't mean we were going to go to bed. He said OK. But then he called me just before five o'clock and told me he wanted me to be wearing black lace bikini panties, and I went over to Marshall Fields and bought two pairs!

Feb. 21

John is unbelievable! I have never been so beautifully and completely fucked in my life! We got to his apartment and John locked the door and simply proceeded to strip me right there in the front hall! Then he laid me down on the living room couch and made love to me with his hands and his mouth for what seemed like hours, eating me until I'd had two orgasms and was practically begging him to fuck me while he just laughed at me. But finally he took me into the bedroom and fucked me very slowly and very gently. Oh, God, he's good! Then, for Christ's sake, we had cocktails! I couldn't believe it, like nothing had happened! We were both naked and we sat at opposite ends of the couch and just chatted. It was weird! But after almost an hour John suddenly said, "Come over here," and when I was standing next to him, he said, "Kneel down and put your mouth on me." It didn't even occur to me to say no. It was like an order but such a lovely order! As soon as I touched him he got beautifully hard and he gently stroked my hair while I sucked him. I really wanted him to come in my mouth, which is strange because I usually don't like that, but with John it seemed natural. But he stopped me before he had an orgasm and took me into the bedroom again. And then, oh, God! he just took me. He actually picked me up and put himself inside me while he was still standing! Then he put me down on the bed with him still inside me and later he flipped me over so I was on top of him and those lovely hard hands were on my breasts. Then suddenly I was kneeling on the bed, and he was standing on the floor behind me and fucking me from behind, and when I started to come he put a finger up my ass and laughed at me again when I screamed. At last he took top and he pinned me to the bed on my back. He hooked my legs back with his arms and held me, his hands like vises so I couldn't move a muscle, and he just pounded his cock into me as hard as he could. He's so strong and I was totally helpless, and oh, God, it felt so incredibly good! I came twice more before he did but when he came he screamed, too! Later I figured it out. John had had two orgasms but I had eight! Eight fucking orgasms! I'm bruised and I'm sore and I'm exhausted, and he can do it again whenever he wants. Please let it be soon!

March 6

John took me to the movies and then he took me to bed. I know I used that word before but that's how it is. He just takes me! He doesn't ask me what I want or what I think or how I feel. He just does it. I remember our first date and how he seemed so sure of himself. And it is such a turn-on! Nobody's ever treated me that way before, and I love it. I'm not weak, either mentally or physically, but, it's like I'm a little girl with him. He wiggles his finger and I jump. And oh God! when he puts those iron hands on me and holds me down on the bed I just go lovely limp. God! I wonder where it goes from here? I can't wait to find out. But I'm scared, too.

March 21

I haven't seen that son of a bitch John for two weeks and now he tells me he's going on a trip to New Orleans! Said he'd send me a postcard! I played it cool on the phone, but I was so fucking mad and frustrated that I cried afterwards.

March 26

I can't believe it! Harry has to go on a trip, too! And I'm going to spend the weekend in New Orleans with John! Whoopee!

April 2

How can I possibly describe the last three days? I don't understand what has happened to me. I'm not even me any more. We got to New Orleans at about eight o'clock Friday night and went right to the hotel. There's a room John always stays in at a little hotel . . . tucked away on a back street in the French Quarter. Actually it's two rooms. There's a tiny living room downstairs and a bedroom upstairs, tucked under the eaves with a huge four-poster bed under a beamed ceiling. By nine o'clock, I was naked and John's hands were on my body again. And in my body. He held me like a bowling ball with his right hand, one finger in my ass and his thumb in my soaking wet cunt, while his left hand was wrapped in my hair holding me flat to the bed while he slowly kissed and licked my belly and breasts and bit my nipples. Somehow he knows just how rough to be and he hurts me just a little, and it all mixes in with the lovely pleasure that I get from that raw strength.

Afterward we went out and walked over to to Mississippi River. John told me he wanted to show me something. We walked along the river for a way and finally we came to a little sort of platform and John told me it marked the place where they used to sell slaves. John was standing behind me and he took one of my wrists in each hand and pulled my arms behind me and held them there. And then he asked me if I'd like to be his slave! I started to kid him but he squeezed my wrists and I shut up. Then he turned me around, still holding both my hands behind me with just one of his and he put his other hand under my chin and forced me to look at him. "Give yourself to me for the weekend," he said. I asked him for what and he said, "For anything I want."

It was like he was looking inside me. I tried to look away but he pulled my head back and he said it again. "Give yourself to me for the weekend." I couldn't speak, and I think that if John hadn't been holding me I would have sunk down on my knees. "Give yourself to me, Marsha," he said again. Finally I answered and I told him I was afraid to. He caught my hair in his hand and pulled my head back. I closed my eyes. "Look at me," he said, like an order. I opened my eyes and looked at him and that tore it. My whole gut had turned to soup and was leaking out of my cunt. I could hardly breathe and there were tears running down my cheeks even though I wasn't crying. "Give yourself to me," he said again, almost in a growl this time. I slumped against him and I whispered, "Yes, yes," into his chest. And God help me, I meant it! There was absolutely nothing I wouldn't have done for him and nothing that I wouldn't have let him do to me.

The rest of the weekend is a lovely warm moist blur. I was being led by a master dancer through the most intricate and erotic of dance routines, choreographed just for his pleasure but resulting inevitably in my pleasure as well. For example, right there on that little slave platform, after I'd committed myself to him, John ordered me to strip to the waist and I removed my blouse and bra with absolutely no thought or hesitation. John turned me around so that I could look out onto the river and he stood behind me with his arms around me, his fingers playing with my nipples. I was almost disappointed when he didn't hurt them. Later that night he ordered me to kneel next to him and suck his cock until he came in my mouth and when he did I said, "Thank you" and I said it again an hour later after he had come again, this time in my cunt.

The next morning we took a shower together and he washed my pussy and then bent me over and took me from behind while the water poured down on my head, soaking my hair, and when I yelled, "Oh shit!" he said he was going to wash my mouth out for talking dirty and he covered his cock with soap and made me suck it. Afterwards he handed me a towel and had me dry him, kneeling to do his legs and feet. He spent all day Saturday showing me "his town" and I loved it. We were like two kids, laughing and holding hands and carrying drinks from Pat O'Brien's down the street. I almost forgot our agreement but late that afternoon we stopped in a Woolworth store and John bought some clothesline. I asked John what it was for and he said, "To tie you up with," like it was the most natural thing in the world, and suddenly everything inside of me sort of shifted and I felt the heat and the tingle spreading up from my cunt. We had a lovely late dinner at Antoine's, and then strolled Bourbon Street and had Irish coffee at some little place and just listened to some jazz. I tried to concentrate but I couldn't really. Half of me wanted so desperately to go back to the hotel while the other half wanted to run away. Finally, at about midnight, John put his hand on my arm and just said, "Now," and he got up and walked out and I followed him, walking behind him all the way back to the hotel. He never looked back, just assuming that I was there.

First he made love to me, and for the first time he was gentle all the way through. I kept waiting for those hands to dig into my body but they never did. And then he took the clothesline and tied me standing at the foot of the bed, my legs spread and my ankles tied to the bed legs and my wrists tied high to the massive end posts. I can't believe now that I let him do it but I didn't even think of fighting him. When he had finished, I asked him if he was going to hurt me and he said that he didn't know, but that it didn't make any difference because I had given myself to him for absolutely anything he might want. He was so matter-of-fact that I didn't even think of answering. Then he went and took a shower and brushed his teeth and went to bed and read for a while, and finally he turned off the light.

I couldn't believe it! I started to ask him how long he intended to leave me there, but before I could even begin he told me to shut up and I did. I just stood there. It didn't hurt at first. As a matter of fact, it was almost comfortable. But after an hour or more I began to get tired and one leg started to cramp and I had to sort of hang from my wrists to take the weight off it. Finally it began to hurt for real. My wrists were being scraped by the rope and the muscles in my legs were on fire. But I was terrified of what might happen if I woke John up, and so I just tried to stand it and it was getting light outside before I finally broke down and began to cry. That woke John up and he got out of bed and untied me and took me into the bed and held me in his arms and went back to sleep. And I just lay there with my lips against his shoulder and whispered, "Thank you, thank you," over and over again.

Sunday morning we had breakfast at Brennan's and John introduced me to his friend, Tony, who was a Captain. But I couldn't believe how he did it. "Marsha, this is Tony," he said, and then, "Tony, this is my slave, Marsha." Tony didn't even bat an eye, and when he came back to take our order he didn't even look at me. Instead he took John's order and then, still looking at John, he asked, "And what will your slave have?" and John ordered for me.

On the way home on the plane, John asked the stewardess for a blanket, and after he spread it over both our laps he ordered me to masturbate him. I did it for nearly an hour. He never came. But I did.

Now I'm home alone and I've been writing this for almost an hour. And I still can't believe it all really happened. And I'm so mixed up!

And I'm afraid, too. But even that's mixed up. I'm afraid that sooner or later John is going to really hurt me. But I'm even more afraid that I might not see him again.

I'm so fucked up!

April 11

I'm John's slave! What else can I say? We went to his apartment and cooked dinner together, and afterward he sat on the couch and told me to kneel in front of him and then he just talked to me. First he said that he understood that I loved Harry just like he loved his wife and that he didn't want to break up my marriage. But then he said that whenever we were together he wanted it to be the way it had been in New Orleans. He told me how much pleasure it gave him to have a woman give herself to him like I had done and he told me that he'd had other women that way before, back when he used to live in New York. And then he told me that he thought it would be good for me, too, and he asked if New Orleans had been as exciting for me as it had been for him, and I nodded my head yes.

Then he handed me a little gift-wrapped box and told me to open it. Inside was a very plain, wide brass arm band with the initials "J Q" engraved on it. John told me that if I accepted the band and put it on, it would mean that I would be his slave and that he would own me completely whenever we were together. I finally got up the courage to speak and I asked him what I'd have to do if I was his slave, and he said, "Anything I want. Anything that gives me pleasure." And then I asked him if I was his slave, would he ever whip me and he said, "Of course." Just like that. "Of course." I asked if that would be to punish me if I didn't obey him and he said yes, but then he said, "But I also will whip you because it will give me pleasure. It won't make any difference if you've been obedient or not."

It took a while for that to sink in. Finally I asked him, "In other words, if I agree to be your slave there will be times when you will whip me just for fun?" He nodded yes and then I asked, "How hard?" and he said, "As hard as I feel like." I couldn't believe how matter-of-fact he was. I was still kneeling in front of him and I was just staring at the arm band. Finally John reached out and gently lifted my head and those goddamn eyes of his looked at me and I couldn't look away. Then he started talking to me very softly and gently. He re-

minded me of the night I'd spent tied to the foot of the bed in New Orleans and he told me that he knew it had hurt me but that it had given him a tremendous amount of pleasure and excitement to go to sleep with me there, knowing I'd still be there whenever he woke up. And he said that despite the pain, he knew it had been exciting for me, too. And then he told me that that was how it would always be when we were together . . . that he'd do whatever gave him pleasure but that it would give me pleasure, too. Even the pain. And finally he told me that just as I could decide to be his slave I could also decide not to be his slave, and that all I would have to do would be to give the arm band back to him. But he also explained that I would only be able to do that once and that if I ever did give it back to him, he would let me go but that I'd never see him again.

I just knelt there looking at him and at the arm band and then John picked it up and held it out to me. And then he said, "I want you to give yourself to me, Marsha. I want you to be my slave." He stopped talking for a second, and then he added, "But if you can't do it, I want you to leave and we won't see each other again." I didn't do anything for maybe two minutes. I was numb and I was so scared I was actually trembling. But suddenly, almost in a kind of flash, I knew that there was no way in the world that I could walk out of there and never feel those hands on me again, and without thinking any more I nodded my head and reached out and took the arm band out of his hand and put it on my right arm. And then I looked up at him. "Who are you?" he asked me and I said, "I'm Marsha." And then he said,"What are you," and I said, "I'm your slave." And from the bottom of my heart I meant it, and I reached out and took John's hand and kissed it.

The first order John gave me was to go into the bedroom and strip and lie on the bed. He waited almost half an hour before he came in and all the time I just lay there without moving a muscle. And after he'd made love to me I said, "Thank you," and he slapped me on the face ever so lightly and said, "From now on it's 'thank you, Sir.' " "Thank you, Sir," I repeated like a little kid.

Or, come to think of it, like an obedient slave.

April 25

I have a slave collar to go with my arm band! Actually it's a short length of heavy steel chain with a heavy steel padlock. I met John at the apartment after work, and as soon as I got there he ordered me to kneel and then he put the chain around my neck and fastened it with the padlock and put the key in his pocket. Then he told me we were going out to dinner. I asked him what people would think and he said, "Who cares?" Actually I don't think anyone noticed and I was sort of disappointed. I know it's crazy but I almost want people to know what I am to John. I'm proud to be his slave. After dinner another surprise. John had fastened another short piece of chain to the head of his bed and he ordered me to strip and lie on the bed and then he locked the two chains together. Then he went out and watched TV. And, oh, God, how can I explain how it felt to lie there, chained to John's bed, just waiting for him to come back and do whatever it was he was going to do. I was scared silly. But I've never felt so alive in my life! And when he finally did come back and began to make love to me, I came almost immediately and screamed and John laughed at me. And later I just hugged him and whispered, "Thank you, Sir," over and over again, and when he finally unlocked the chain from my neck I felt sad.

May 2

The whole world is out of focus and I'm just pretending to be me. I have a date with John tomorrow night and this morning, almost as soon as I got into my office, John called me. He said, "Good morning, slave," and I said, "Good morning, Sir," and then he said, "I just thought you'd like to know in advance that I plan to whip you tomorrow night." And then he just hung up!

And I've been trembling inside ever since. Partly because I'm scared. But mostly because I'm so turned on I don't think I can stand another minute of waiting. I made myself come twice in the ladies' room at the office, and I've done it twice more tonight and I'm praying that Harry will want to make love when he gets home. But I know it won't help.

I don't know how I'm going to get through the day tomorrow. And, of course, I have no idea how I'm going to get through tomorrow night!

Oh God, I hope I don't scream!

May 3

I didn't scream! And my body has the marks of John's whip and I love them and I'm so goddamn proud of myself!

When I got to the apartment, John was already there and there was a pair of handcuffs hanging by a chain from one of the ceiling rings where the planters usually hang. (I don't know why I never before guessed their true purpose.)

I knelt and kissed John's hand, and then he asked me if I remembered what he'd told me on the phone yesterday and I whispered, "Yes, Sir," and he said, "Good," and that whenever I was ready I should strip and go over and put the handcuffs on myself. I didn't hesitate for even a second. I took off my clothes as fast as I could, and walked over and raised my arms and snapped the handcuffs on my wrists. My hands were several inches above my head but my feet were flat on the floor.

John came over and put his hands on my breasts and asked me if I knew what was going to happen, and I said, "Yes, Sir," and he asked me what and I said, "You're going to whip me," and then he asked if I knew why I was going to be whipped and I said, "Because it will make you happy," and he said that was right, and then he put a blindfold on me, and oh God, my insides were leaking out of me!

First he played with me and used the whip to sort of caress me all over my body for several minutes until I knew he could see my body trembling, and then all of a sudden there was the sharp searing pain of the whip across my ass followed by two more, very quickly, across my back, and I jumped and cried, "Oh!" but by then the whip was caressing me again.

He whipped me maybe fifty times, but they were spaced out so that the pain of each one was isolated, almost as if John wanted me to be able to feel and think about each stroke of the whip all by itself. And in between those bright white-hot miniseconds of pain that same whip stroked my ass and my belly and my nipples while my mind wondered where the whip would land the next time and my body grew almost impatient waiting for it to strike again.

The last two were very hard, one across each breast, and I cried out again, but not loudly, and then John's fingers were suddenly inside me and my orgasm was immediate and monumental.

Later John chained me to the bed and carefully traced all the welts with his tongue before he fucked me, and he told me how beautiful they were.

He's right. They are *beautiful. They make my body beautiful and they prove that I really do belong to him. And I can't wait for him to whip me again.*

And, God help me, I've changed my mind. Now I want him to make me scream!

June 13

Without my realizing it, my relationship with John has slowly become more and more intense. I don't know whether he planned it that way or if we've just let it happen together. He owns me completely. There is absolutely no question about that. His chains and his whip are a natural part of my life, and there's been a subtle shift so that now the times that we aren't together are make-believe. It's the times that I spend in helpless bondage, waiting for him to use me, that make up the real world now.

He whips me at least a little almost every time we are together. That's become natural, too. And I always try to take as much as I possibly can and not cry, but sometimes I do. That's when John usually asks me to say, "Please stop." He wants to make me beg. But so far I have resisted. Instead, I always answer, "I'm your slave. You can do whatever you want," even though I know that eventually I'll probably begin screaming, at least a little, and I usually do.

We both know that sooner or later John will "break" me, and I'll be forced to beg, but it's like a game and he's taking me so slowly down the road that so far I've managed to keep up. I'm so proud of how much pain I can take and how much pleasure I give to him that way, and I know that John is proud of me, too.

And always after the whipping comes the reward of his hands and his body. I've never had an orgasm while John was whipping me but God! how ready I get and I usually come immediately, and sometimes he makes me come the first time while I'm still tied up, and what an incredible feeling that is!

But always John ends the evening with what I think of to myself as his "power fuck" and his hands hold me helpless while his body tears into mine, and I know now that that's what it's all about and I also know that if he ever stopped whipping me it wouldn't be as good.

And just writing that down suddenly made something clear. I actually need the whipping now. The pain and the pleasure are inseparable for me, one leading to and making the other possible.

I'm not sure that's good. But that's the way it is.

July 11

It's the 3-month anniversary of the day I became John's slave. I bought him a beautiful riding crop as a present and of course John used it on me. God, it hurts! . . . an awful, sharp, cutting pain . . . particularly when John uses it on the inside of my thighs. But it leaves the most beautiful marks that last much longer than the others.

But I've got to be careful. Harry asked me the other day how come I was still wearing long pajamas in July. Thank goodness we usually make love with the lights out!

July 30

Three weeks ago John decided he wanted to fuck me in the ass. He has often had a finger in me there and I could handle that. It was even sexy. But on the night he decided, he put two fingers in me and it hurt a little. But he's determined, and he's been working on me. What's even more incredible is that I've been working on myself! He's slowly stretched me with dildos and now I'm sitting here with a medium-size "butt plug" in me. John has ordered me to have it in me for at least two hours every night and it's weird sitting here watching TV with Harry and feeling it there inside me. It's almost as if John is here fucking me but he's invisible and Harry can't see him.

And next week John says I'm going to have to start wearing it in the office!

There's no part of my body that belongs to me any more. And I don't care.

Aug. 9

My Master has finally made me beg. Not with his whip but with his cock.

Yesterday I put a new, even larger butt plug in my ass and I went to work and left it there all day. After work I met John at the Drake Hotel and we had dinner at his private club, and he told me how turned on he was knowing it was there. All during dinner he was gentle with me, as if he was taking care of me, and I knew that it was going to happen that night.

Finally we went back to the apartment, and John very carefully undressed me and then he tied me kneeling, bent over the bench he has at the end of his bed. He tied my hands behind me but used a strap through my collar to keep me from straightening up. He had me suck him until he was hard, and then he moved behind me and had me put KY jelly on his cock. When he was ready, he carefully removed the butt plug and then he whispered, "I love you, slave," and then I felt his cock beginning to move into my ass.

I don't think his cock is bigger around than the butt plug. Maybe longer. But I was suddenly terrified and I must have tensed because it hurt more than anything John's ever done to me. Even when only the tip was inside me, it felt like I was being torn apart and I screamed, but he slowly kept moving it deeper into me and that's when I came apart completely and begged him to stop but of course he didn't. At least not for long. He pulled his cock out of me and went and got a gag, and I just kept begging, "Please don't! . . . please don't!" until he slapped me and forced the gag into my mouth and strapped it tight. Then he went into me again. Oh, God! it hurt so terribly and I screamed and screamed into the gag, but he just kept going and finally his cock was all the way inside my ass, and it felt so huge and it felt like something must have torn open.

At first he didn't move, but then he slowly began to fuck me, pulling his cock back just a little and then forcing it back into me again, and each time I screamed. But then I heard John's voice and he was almost growling and he was saying something like, "Oh, God, I love doing this to you. God, I love fucking my slave in the ass," and it was like he was talking to himself. But somehow hearing him made me relax a little or something because it stopped hurting quite so much, and John must have felt it because he leaned over and loosened the gag and then he began to really fuck me and although it still hurt I could handle it, and that's when John asked me who I was and I answered, "I'm your slave," and then he asked me what I felt, and I answered, "I feel my Master's cock fucking me in the ass," and as soon as I'd said that John pumped his cock into me very hard and very fast a couple of times and I screamed again but so did he, and then he came in my ass.

Afterward John cleaned me and there was some blood, and when I saw it I started to cry and for the first time ever John told me he was sorry. I didn't say anything but I went and got one of the whips and I came back to him and handed him the whip and I knelt in front of him and I said, "Don't be sorry. I'm your slave and you can do anything to me that you want." Then I apologized for begging and told him that I wanted him to whip me as punishment for being so weak, and that I wanted him to fuck me in the ass again as soon as possible so that I could make it up to him.

That's when he hugged me, and although I'm not sure, I think he was crying too and I just hugged him back and kept telling him how much I loved him and loved being his slave.

Aug. 27

Another long weekend with John . . . this time in Miami. We stayed in a lovely huge suite at the Fountainbleu and just had a ball! We played golf and swam and lay in the sun and went to a marvelous restaurant where John knew the maitre d' and visited a beautiful old mansion called Viscaya.

John didn't even whip me for the first two days. He just took care of me and we made love maybe four or five times a day. Christ, he's like a teenager sometimes! I was beginning to wonder if he was going soft on me. No chance! Sunday morning he made love to me and we went to breakfast and then back to the room. Then John proceeded to whip me for close to an hour, using the riding crop and very carefully whipping my entire body until I was completely covered with bright red stripes that were no more than an inch apart anywhere on me. Then he put my chain collar on my neck and told me to put on a bikini and my full-length beach "cover up" and then he took me down to the pool.

And then the son of a bitch ordered me to take off the robe and lie there on a sun chair where everyone could see. God, it was wild! People just stared and two old ladies got up and moved away and a waiter actually dropped a tray full of drinks, and John and I just sat there acting perfectly normal. I was horribly embarrassed at first, but then it started to be funny, especially when we heard some little girl ask her mommy if I was a zebra, and we started taking turns seeing how outrageous we could be. At one point I got up and slowly walked all the way around the pool and later John asked some lady to take a picture of the two of us together, telling her that we wanted to have one to show the kids when we got home.

Finally we went back up to the suite, but I got in the last shot by removing my robe in the elevator when another couple got in and they almost died. We made love and giggled the rest of the afternoon and John whipped me all over again just before we went to dinner, but this time I wore a long dress because John said that he wanted to be the only one who knew that my body was covered with the marks of his whip.

God, I have such a wonderful Master!

Sept. 16

My Master has been away for three weeks on a combined business trip and vacation with his family. For three weeks I have not felt his whip on my body, or felt his cock inside my cunt or my ass, or felt those marvelously cruel hands that turn me to warm syrup so easily. God, I miss them all so much.

Sept. 20

I'm so proud of myself! I decided I wanted to give John a coming-home present, so I called him at work and told him I had a surprise for him and that if it was OK with him I'd like to meet him at the apartment. The way I explained it he thought I was going to cook him dinner.

But instead I got there early and I laid out all the whips and put the leather cuffs on my wrists and ankles and hung a sign around my neck that said, "Welcome Home, Master." Then I pulled the hassock over under the ceiling rings and stood on it. I chained my ankles together and put the gag and blindfold on myself and a clothespin on each nipple. And finally I fastened my wrists to the ceiling rings and waited for John to come home.

Fortunately I didn't have to wait very long, and when I heard his key in the lock I kicked away the hassock so that John found me there naked and hanging by my wrists.

The longest I've ever hung that way until today was maybe about five minutes but this time it must have been much longer. John didn't say a word, but I heard him stop in front of me and then he went into the bathroom and finally I heard him getting a beer out of the refrigerator. I wanted so badly for him to say something or touch me or whip me but I just hung there and it really began to hurt.

But finally, just as I was afraid I was going to begin to scream, I felt his hands touch me and then he removed the clothespins from my nipples and kissed each one. I heard him whisper, "I love you, slave, very very much," and then he moved the hassock back so I could stand on it and he took me down and took me into the bedroom and made love to me very gently. And all the time he kept telling me how much he loved me and how wonderful my present had been, and I was so happy and proud that I thought I was going to cry.

Afterward we went out to the A&P and bought some food and cooked dinner together, and all the time John was gentle and loving and sweet and it was really nice, but it finally got on my nerves and so after dinner I asked him to hang me up by my wrists again and whip me. He did, until I screamed, but he didn't stop and it turned out to be the hardest beating he's ever given me. And when he finally took me down again he made me blow him and then he fucked me in the ass, and finally he chained me to the bed and fucked me as hard and as brutally as he's ever done.

I know he was deliberately mean, and that he went out of his way to hurt me even more than he usually does. But I also know even more than I ever did that he really does love me very, very much. Finally, we both know that I asked for it because I wanted it to happen, and, even more important, because I needed it to happen.

Being John's slave was no longer in any way just a matter of my being what John wants me to be. Now it is entirely a matter of being what I want me to be.

Oct. 21

I'm pregnant! I have been for seven weeks. Harry is ecstatic. Thank God it's his and not John's. But oh, God, what will I do?

Nov. 6

I have asked John for my freedom and he has given it to me. At first we had planned to have dinner and make love one more time, but then John decided that might not be a good idea. I think he was right, although I would have loved feeling his body on and in mine one more time. But I met him for lunch instead and I returned the arm band to him. John said that I could keep it if I wanted to but I told him that I'd better not. Actually, I knew that I wouldn't have been able to bear looking at it after we were apart.

After lunch I didn't go back to work but I came home. It's al-

most nine o'clock now and Harry won't be home for another hour, but that's just as well, because maybe I'll stop crying by then.

• • •

Jan. 6 [Three years later]

I have made Xerox copies of my journal and I'm sending them to John for his book, and for the first time ever I'm writing something in it that I know someone else will read.

My little girl, Cindy, is two and a half years old now. She's beautiful and she's bright and I'm so very glad we have her, and now Harry and I are trying to arrange for her to have a brother or sister.

Seeing John again was such a shock! It had been so long and what with carrying Cindy and then having her, I got over him much better than I ever thought I would. But when I suddenly saw him standing there at the bar, it was like an electric jolt. But he's so smart! He started to reach out to shake my hand but then he pulled his hand back, so he never actually touched me.

There's a song in Porgy and Bess *where Bess begs Porgy to keep the bad guy, Crown, away from her and she sings, "don't let him touch me with those hot hands," because she knows that if Crown touches her she won't be able to control herself.*

I think it's that way with me. I pray that John will stay away from me. I know that if he ever touched me the way he used to, I'd be right back where I was. His slave.

And I also know that I'd never have the strength to ask for my freedom again.

15

"Golden Moments"

I have a friend named Tim who, with his lovely submissive wife, Sandy, lives in the wilds of Wisconsin. I have had Sandy as my slave on numerous occasions and Tim and I have shared many good times.

When he heard about this book, Tim told me, "Don't forget to include some 'Golden Moments.'" I asked Tom what he meant and he said, "You know . . . those special little times where everything is either so perfect or so exciting or so much fun or so meaningful that it sort of all by itself is what S/M is all about."

As an example, Tim told me about having once taken Sandy out into the woods on a summer night, stripping her, and tying her spread-eagled between two trees. He whipped her gently for a while and made love to her with his mouth and hands and then he left her there, telling her that when he came back he was going to whip her much more severely. The idea, of course, was to let Sandy stay there, tied and naked and all alone in the night, thinking about what was coming.

But Tim didn't want Sandy to get too scared, so he started back after only an hour or so. He walked quietly and when he got back to where he had left Sandy, he found her with her head thrown back and her eyes closed, sort of hanging by her wrists, with almost a smile on her face.

He touched Sandy, who jumped and opened her eyes. Then she

frowned slightly and whispered, "You came back too soon."

"In what way?" Tim asked her.

"I wasn't completely terrified yet," Sandy answered.

That was a "Golden Moment" for Tim.

The following are some of mine.

ISABELLE

It was a bright spring morning when I woke up in my Chicago apartment with a brand-new slave, Isabelle, with whom, the night before, I had shared a very long first meeting.

Isabelle is a very special kind of person. She is, in my opinion, a "Classic O" type, but with one very major difference. For her there is no "Sir Stephen." Instead, Isabelle describes herself as an "independent submissive," and as such she travels all over the country, spending time with a whole series of "Masters" . . . a weekend in Los Angeles with Dave . . . the following weekend in Boston with Peter . . . and the next weekend in New York with Scott.

Perhaps Isabelle wouldn't agree with me, but I somehow have the feeling that she is not necessarily "independent" by choice. Instead, I think that if Isabelle ever met her *real* Sir Stephen, she would joyfully give up her independence.

I have been with Isabelle several times, but that first evening had been very difficult for her. Like many submissives, Isabelle often fantasized beyond her own real limits, never expecting those fantasies to come true. But this time she had put some of those fantasies into a letter to me without realizing that, unlike so many of her other gentler Masters, I was perfectly capable of making them come to life.

And I had done just that, for almost five hours!

But now it was morning and I had just awakened in bed with Isabelle. I had originally intended to have her sleep on the floor next to my bed, chained to a ring, but I had changed my mind. At any rate, I rolled over and discovered Isabelle kneeling next to me. She was bent low with her head down, her eyes closed, and her arms stretched out in front of her with her wrists crossed. She looked very lovely.

But there was one other small point. On each of her nipples was a particularly painful clamp.

Isabelle felt me roll over but she didn't move. I watched her for a while and then I spoke to her. "What are you doing, slave?" I asked.

"I'm practicing taking pain for you," Isabelle said."

"Why?"

"Because you are very severe and I don't want to disappoint you."

"How long have you been there?" I asked.

"I don't know," Isabelle answered. "Maybe half an hour."

I leaned over and kissed her and then lay back and dozed off again. And when I woke up almost an hour later, Isabelle was still there, practicing taking pain for her new Master.

RACHEL

Rachel was a novice. She was a young, pushy little copywriter at an advertising agency in Chicago, only twenty-four years old but very confident of who she was and where she was going. We had dated and made love several times, and with both of us being so self-assured, our lovemaking had been very good and a lot of fun.

But we had also talked about my "second life" as a dominant and finally, despite her very strong-willed personality, Rachel had decided to experiment by submitting herself to me. She was blindfolded and tied spread-eagled on her bed, her body stretched tight by heavy woven luggage straps tied to her wrists and ankles.

I had teased her sexually for quite a while and she had had an orgasm. Now I was whipping her lightly with my belt across her legs, stomach, and breasts. She began to strain at her bonds, and her breath became fast and shallow as she built toward another orgasm. She screamed a little when she came, and then I began whipping her again. As I did, Rachel spoke for the first time. "Oh, God," she whispered.

"Oh, God, what?" I asked.

Rachel strained at her bonds again, arching her back. "Oh, God, if you only knew how hard it is for me to be submissive, you'd realize what a fucking super prize you've got."

I pulled the blindfold aside to let her look at me. "I know what a fucking super prize I've got," I told her.

And then I replaced the blindfold and began whipping her again . . . a little harder now . . . while my fingers started her toward yet another orgasm.

AMY

Taking a woman as a new slave is always very special. But when a new slave writes a letter as beautiful as the one Amy wrote me after our first encounter, it is, all in itself, a "Golden Moment."

Dear Sir John,

My name is Amy. I am a slave. My Master is Sir John Q_____. He may do anything to me he chooses. I will do whatever he asks of me."
These words were quickly memorized. I hope to understand and accept them just as quickly. I have also memorized the three "slave positions" you taught me and have begun to practice them.

"Master." What a beautiful and unique word! For the first time in my life I saw a real Master; a leader without hesitation; one so sure of his mental, emotional, and physical demands that he conveys his wishes with a glance, a snap of fingers, or a short command and they are instantly obeyed. How could one not do so? I find in you, Sir John, a power so strong! There is power in your glance, touch, tone. A power that demands instant obedience from one who is proud of the opportunity to serve you.

It was so important to me that you approve of me, of my actions, and my ability to learn quickly what you taught me. How fortunate for this slave to have found someone willing to take the time to train her properly. I will sincerely attempt to be one of your best students.

Being beaten with various types of whips and crops was a new experience for me. Each blow found a body tense in anticipation and was exquisite torture. With each blow my insides screamed, "No more! Please! Please!" However, a small chord deep within me would not allow the words to come out. I knew it would eventually end and that you were experienced enough to gauge when that should be. I was proud of me for not spoiling the pleasure you were receiving.

Surely you were aware of how my body trembled the entire time and how often I leaned against something for support as I felt my knees buckle—all because of pain, fear, and the realization that this was real, not a game. I am a slave, Sir John, and you are my Master. My only responsibility is to do your biddings and do them as you expect . . . quickly, questionless, and grateful to you for constantly reinforcing my new role in life by reminding me of just who and what you are and what I am, and for permitting me to serve you.

My head has been saying, "What are you doing? What are you deliberately walking into?" There is a neon sign on a door shouting DANGER, but I am totally committed to walking to that door, passing through, and then, on my knees, moving to my place, kneeling before you, and waiting to serve you and pleasure you in whatever manner you choose. Your will becomes mine. Decisions are yours—and this is such a relief since it is the opposite of my everyday life which requires constant decisions, movement, and communication. This, too, as the pain, is a totally new experience for me . . . the total giving over of my will to another person. God! What an incredibly exquisite pleasure and luxury that is!

Your slave believes you are one of the few men in the world who is not afraid to get what he wants, regardless of society's mores. I pledge myself to serving you obediently and quickly and have great hopes of becoming a slave of whom you are proud, both in private and in public. I know who and what I am and, most important, who you are, what to expect and what is expected of me. I fervently pray that I may serve and please you.

most humbly,

amy

Amy provided me with a second "Golden Moment."

It was the night of Amy's public initiation, and I had arranged to take her to a party at the "Club O" in New York. I had also arranged for her to be the "door prize" for the evening.

Very simply, shortly after arriving at the club at about 10:00 P.M., Amy was stripped and tied to a special "bondage chair" in the middle of the dance floor. The chair was built along the lines of the old stocks, and Amy was forced to kneel on the padded bench with her arms tied securely to each side, while her head was strapped in place so that it protruded at about waist height through a special opening in the back of the chair.

Above her head was posted a sign. It read, "Free Expert Blow Job. For Permission, See Sir John Q." (This was before the advent of AIDS.)

I carry calling cards which simply have "Sir John Q____" engraved on them. During the evening, as various male guests made their requests for my approval, I would grant them permission by giving them one of my cards with, "OK–J.Q." written on it. Two "assistant slaves," Betsy and George, stood watch over Amy while I participated in the party, making sure that no one molested her and that only those men with official permission were "serviced."

After an hour or so, during which time I had handed out perhaps a dozen cards, I stopped by to make sure all was well. That's when I broke up. There was Amy, still properly tied, having just finished swallowing the rewards of her latest customer. George was standing next to her, patting her head. But it was Betsy who got to me. She had once worked in a theater, and as the next "customer" stepped up, Betsy very formally took the calling card, inspected it to make sure it was properly endorsed, and then carefully tore it in half, putting one half in a box next to her and giving the "stub" back to the gentleman, who gave her a sort of bewildered look before stepping forward for his "expert blow job."

Betsy looked up and saw me standing there, grinning at her, and she grinned back. "Shit, Sir John," she said. "You have to keep things organized."

And then she looked back at the several men standing in front of her, all holding cards. "Please keep the line straight," I heard her call out as I went back to the party.

BETTY

Betty was being "trained" and she had been gently disciplined until nearly midnight. When I finally went to bed, I ordered her to kneel next to the bed with her hands behind her and to remain that way in case I should wake up and want to "use" her. I had told her she was to remain there until 4:00 A.M.; if by that time I had not awakened, she could lie down and sleep on the floor by my bed. There was a digital clock with a night light next to my bed where she could see it.

Much later something woke me up. I realized it was Betty, crying quietly. Without letting her know I was awake, I opened one eye. The clock told me it was six minutes before 4:00 and Betty was still kneeling there. But she was obviously in considerable pain: her head was thrown back, her eyes were closed, and there were tears running down her cheeks. Her hands were still behind her but she was continuously moving her body, shifting her weight from one knee to the other in an effort to relieve her terrible discomfort. After all, she had been kneeling there for nearly four hours!

I watched her, not letting her know that I was awake. I remember how beautiful she looked to me with her long hair partially covering one shoulder, her hands behind her, and her breasts thrust toward me. And I remember thinking how much she must love me to be obeying me this way despite her pain and despite the fact that, as far as she knew, I was still sound asleep and couldn't have known if she had chosen to disobey me.

Finally, when four o'clock came, Betty let out a soft cry, lay down next to my bed, and curled up on the small blanket I'd left there for her.

I went back to sleep and I dreamed of her. Next morning, when I found Betty still sleeping there on the floor, I woke her, ordered her into my bed, and made very long and very gentle love to her, telling her how much I loved her.

KATY

Katy had been around the scene for some years and now she was with me. I knew she'd had many experiences with a lot of other dominants, but she still was not, in my opinion, really "experienced." So I had gone out of my way to carefully and privately teach her how to be instantly obedient, subjecting her to immediate punishment at the slightest infraction or hesitation.

Once I felt Katy understood totally what I required of her and that she was prepared to obey those requirements, I took her to an S/M party to "test" her.

We had a lovely time. Two of Katy's former Masters were there, and they properly acknowledged her new status. With the training I'd given her, there was never even a second when she wasn't responding to, and even anticipating, my every wish and need. In short, our relationship had reached that rare point where her response and obedience were so spontaneous that there was never any need to push it. It was just a natural part of everything we did.

I think we both understood how special the evening had been, but when we got back to my apartment Katy confirmed it. After I had taken a shower, Katy was drying me with a huge towel, kneeling in front of me to dry my lower legs and feet. When she finished, she spoke to me, still kneeling.

"May I speak, Master?" she asked.

"Yes," I said.

"May I also look at you, Sir?"

Again I gave my permission. Still kneeling there, Katy reached up, put her hands on the outside of my thighs, bent her head to kiss the tip of my cock, and then, looked up at me. "I just wanted to tell you something very important," she said.

"What's that?"

"I just wanted to tell you that for the first time in my life I finally know what a *real* Master is."

GAYLE

Gayle had always had a fantasy about being kidnapped and sold into slavery.

On a trip to Las Vegas I made that fantasy come true.

During the first two days of our trip I made it a habit to leave Gayle naked and chained loosely to the bed in our hotel room whenever I had to go out alone. This had happened five or six times, so when late Sunday afternoon I told Gayle that I was going out to get an ice cream cone, she wasn't surprised when I locked one end of the long chain onto her ankle and fastened the other end to the foot of the bed.

But twenty minutes later something very different happened!

The door to the room opened suddenly and two very big, rough-looking men came in, closing the door behind them. One of them walked directly over to Gayle, grabbed her by the hair, pulled her head back, and asked her what her name was. When Gayle didn't answer right away, he slapped her across the face and asked her again. This time she managed to whisper, "I'm Gayle."

The man nodded and then produced a key, unlocked the chain, and ordered Gayle to get dressed. As soon as she was ready, the two men, one on each side, took her roughly by the arms, escorted her out of the rear exit of the hotel and across the parking lot to a station wagon. There they quickly handcuffed her hands behind her, blindfolded her, roughly shoved her into the rear deck, and threw a blanket over her.

Then came a forty-five minute drive, the last fifteen minutes over rather rough roads, which left no doubt in Gayle's mind that they were well out in the country. When at last the ride ended, Gayle, still handcuffed and blindfolded, was taken from the car and led into a house, where the men removed her handcuffs and ordered her to strip. The blindfold was removed only after she had been chained to a vertical rack. Then, just before leaving her alone, one of the men pulled Gayle's head up and stared at her for a few seconds. Finally he shook his head and muttered, "Christ! I'm sure as hell glad I'm not you!"

Gayle was naked, so tautly suspended by the chains on her wrists that just the tips of toes touched the floor. Moreover, as she looked around, she discovered that she was in a large, fully equipped, sound-proofed torture chamber. She was left there alone for close to an hour!

Finally the door to the chamber opened and a powerfully built, stern-looking Mistress, dressed entirely in studded black leather and carrying a riding crop, entered. She stood in front of Gayle, looking at her for a while before suddenly swinging the riding crop across Gayle's breasts.

"Pay attention, slave!" she ordered in a slightly accented voice. "Your Master, John Q, has had a misfortune. Two nights ago he lost almost twenty-three thousand dollars in a poker game. Unfortunately, he could not pay. Consequently, instead of payment, he has given you to me for the rest of the day and night. I am Mistress Joan, and I have invited several extremely wealthy men here who will pay a great deal of money for the privilege of torturing you. There are no limits, except how much they choose to pay."

Mistress Joan stopped talking and studied Gayle for a brief moment. Then she added, "We will begin soon. In the meantime, I suggest you try to rest if you can. It will be a very long and very difficult evening."

Actually, the evening would last about five hours. Gayle was left alone again for a while to allow the tension to build, but after half an hour or so Mistress Joan returned. She explained that, since none of the men wanted to take the chance of being recognized, Gayle would be blindfolded for the rest of the night. As soon as the blindfold was in place, Gayle was unchained from the rack and tied bent forward over a whipping bench.

Ten minutes later, the first customer arrived. In Gayle's presence, he bargained with Mistress Joan, finally agreeing to pay $5,000 in order to whip Gayle for half an hour and then fuck her in the ass. Afterward, he paid an additional $1,000 to have Gayle suck his cock clean.

The second customer did not speak English, and so Mistress Joan translated. Gayle was to be hung by her wrists and the man would pay $100 per stroke to whip her. By the time he was finished, his bill was $10,000.

The third customer wanted to whip only Gayle's breasts. Consequently, a price of $250 per stroke was set, and he whipped her twenty-five times. Then, for an additional $2,500 he was allowed to have Gayle perform oral sex on him until he had a orgasm.

It went that way through a total of six customers who spent a total of $41,000 for Gayle's services. During the entire time Gayle never saw who was whipping her.

Nor did she ever see me sitting quietly in a corner of the chamber, making sure she was not seriously hurt.

After the last "customer" had left, Gayle was chained and left kneeling on the floor for another half hour before finally being redressed, handcuffed, dumped back into the station wagon, and returned to the hotel room where she was stripped and rechained in exactly the same way that I had left her some six hours earlier.

The first "Golden Moment" came when I returned to the room some twenty minutes after Gayle's "abductors" had left. I was, of course, eating an ice cream cone.

I walked over to where Gayle lay on the bed and she looked up at me. "I'm sorry I was gone so long," I said. "Something came up." And then I added, "Anything happen while I was away?"

Despite all that had happened to her during the last long hours, Gayle promptly broke up, laughing until she cried.

The second "Golden Moment" came later that night. I took Gayle to bed and, after we had made very long and very gentle love, Gayle described to me all that had happened to her. She finished by describing how she had been left chained and kneeling after the last customer, waiting to see what would happen next.

"What were you thinking then?" I asked her.

Gayle hugged me. "I was just thinking how goddamn lucky I was to have Sir John for a Master," she said.

DEE

Her name was Dee and she was a little 18-year-old, mostly gay sub-missive when I met her in a "sex shop" in Greenwich Village and invited her to one of my Friday night parties. One of the other expected guests was a husky, blond 23-year-old "switchable" named Sandra, who had been submissive to me for a few months but who was happily bisexual and had always wanted to have a female slave of her own. So I had decided to give Dee to Sandra as a surprise gift.

I had given Dee a brief introductory "training course," teaching her to assume various basic submissive positions on command and explaining to her the proper "manners" of a slave, which included never looking a Master or Mistress in the eye unless specifically ordered to do so. Dee learned quickly and when Sandra arrived Dee knelt before her, kissed her feet, and recited the "litany" I had taught her, acknowledging that she was a slave and would do whatever her new Mistress commanded.

Shortly thereafter, Dee, Sandra, and I, together with two other guests, went across the street for supper. Dee sat next to Sandra, pouring wine for her, lighting her cigarettes, and being generally attentive. All the while, of course, she kept her eyes demurely and obediently downcast. When the waiter came, Sandra ordered for her new slave, deciding that although the rest of us would be having dinner, little Dee would be restricted to a simple salad.

The food was served and the usual conversation ensued, covering all sorts of topics. As was proper, Dee remained silent, her head still slightly bowed, staring down at her plate. But as soon as Sandra had excused herself to go to the ladies room, ordering Dee to remain at the table, Dee let out a huge sigh.

I looked at Dee. Her head was still bent and her eyes still downcast while she very slowly rearranged the salad with her fork. "What's the matter?" I asked her.

Dee continued to look down. "Gosh," she said. "I wish I could look at my Mistress when she speaks to me. She's so beautiful!"

"That's not allowed," I reminded her.

"I know," Dee answered. And then she smiled shyly. "At least there's one thing nice," she added.

"What's that?"

"I'm really getting to know this cucumber awfully well!"

SUSAN

As part of a test, I had done something very painful to Susan. It had been quick but it had hurt her a lot . . . much more than I intended . . . and she had screamed, curled up into a ball, and cried for a long time.

Later, in bed, I talked to Susan about it and she finally told me, with complete honesty, that if she had known at the beginning how severe a Master I could be, she might never have agreed to become my slave.

"But you have the right to leave any time," I reminded her.

"I know."

"And I can't promise that I won't hurt you that badly again," I added.

"I know that, too."

"Then why don't you leave?" I asked her.

Susan rolled over and hugged me. "I've thought about it," she admitted.

"And?"

Susan hugged me again. "And I decided that you really do have the right to do anything to me that you want."

JENNIFER

The first "slave auction" I knew about was held at the old "Les Scenes" club in New York, where a beautiful blonde named Honey acted as the auctioneer. At these auctions, dominants would use scrip to buy a slave for an hour. A certain amount of scrip was provided with each entrance fee, and additional scrip was given for each drink purchased or could be bought for $1.00 for each $1,000 in scrip.

I had brought my slave, Jennifer, a beautiful six-foot-two blonde dancer who, needless to say, drew a lot of attention. She was dressed in a black leotard, her hands were handcuffed, and around her neck was a black leather collar to which my leash was attached.

Six slaves were auctioned that night. The first three were middle-aged submissive men who put themselves up for sale, hoping to be bought and spanked by a dominant woman. They were sold for $5,000 to $10,000 each. The fourth was also male, but he was a handsome, blonde, young gay, very well-built and dressed entirely in leather. He brought a bid of $55,000.

Then a dominant friend of mine put his submissive wife on the block. She was a very good-looking woman, about twenty-eight years old, with a dynamite body, and dressed in a very sexy, provocative, and revealing harem costume. She was sold for $95,000.

Finally it was Jennifer's turn. I led her to the slave block, removed the leash from her collar, and stood back.

Two separate groups of dominants, having heard that Jennifer was to be auctioned, had pooled their scrip, and the bidding went on for a long time. The winning bid was $335,000!

That was a "Golden Moment" all by itself; but the next morning, Jennifer topped it. As was her duty, she brought me orange juice and knelt beside my bed to serve it to me. Then she started to giggle.

"What's so funny, slave?" I asked.

"Oh, I was just thinking about last night's auction," she answered.

"What about it?"

"Well," Jennifer replied, "I was remembering how when the other slaves were auctioned, Honey would say something like, 'Now we're going to sell George,' or 'Now we're going to sell Bryant,' or 'The next slave to be auctioned will be Grace.' "

"So what?" I asked.

"Well," Jennifer continued, "when my turn came, Honey said, 'We are now going to auction Sir John Q's slave, Jennifer.' "

"So what's so funny about that?" I asked.

Jennifer started to giggle again, and then she said, "I just realized that I was the only brand-name slave in the auction."

TINA

My slave, Tina, wrote me this note one night while I was sleeping. If you knew Tina, you would know how very special it was for me and why I will always treasure it.

Dear Master,

I really want to be special for you. I'm sure you already know that. Sometimes I think you are overly concerned about how much you hurt

*me, but I also know that there are some really severe things that you
have always wanted to do to a slave that you would enjoy. Please do
them to me.*

*I understand that I will have to endure a lot of pain, but I accept
whatever happens as the price that must be paid for your pleasure.
I've said this before, but maybe this note will overcome your inhibitions.
I hope it does.*

*It would be wonderful to have you just "take" me, restrain me
completely, and then do all of the things you've ever done to any other
slave plus whatever else would turn you on but that you have never
done to any slave.*

*And so this note is for you to show me when I am helpless to
remind me that I have told you that whatever you do to me is all
right because I belong to you. (As I always say in my "slave pledge,"
you are my Master and you have the right to do anything you want
to me.)*

*I know that because of this note you will do things to me that
I will hate, but this is my "consent form" for you to do* absolutely
anything and everything *to me that will bring you pleasure.*

I love you, Master.

slave tina

URSULA

My slave, Ursula, and I were sitting on the small stage at the back
of the old Hellfire Club one night. Ursula had my chain locked around
her neck; she was also wearing handcuffs and was on a leash.

Despite Ursula's obvious submissive status, a young man approached
us and, totally ignoring me, knelt next to Ursula. Looking up at her
worshipfully, he spoke. The conversation went like this:

Man. "Oh, please, Mistress, may I be your slave?"

Ursula: "No."

Man: "May I just kneel here and adore you?"

Ursula: "No."

Man: "May I kiss that beautiful lock that you're wearing?"

Ursula: "No."

Man: "May I worship your feet?"

Ursula: "No."

Man: "May I lick your boots?"

Ursula: "No."

Man: "Would you whip me?"

Ursula: "No."

Man: "Would you like to use my body as an ash tray?"

Ursula: "No."

Man: "Would you like to crush my balls with the heels of your boots?"

Ursula: "No."

Man: "Could I be your toilet slave?"

Ursula didn't know that he meant that he wanted her to piss or shit on him. All she knew was that when she went to the bathroom her three-year-old son sometimes handed her the toilet paper. And so she answered, "No. My little boy does that for me."

The man immediately stood up. "You're sick!" he yelled at Ursula, and walked away.

MARIE

I was at the Vault, an S/M club in New York, and had done a sexy and exciting scene with my slave, Donna. Donna is blonde and pretty, has an excellent body, and is truly and totally submissive. The scene had lasted close to an hour and the crowd had definitely been turned on.

Shortly after the scene, a nice-looking man came up to me and told me that he was there with his wife, who much very wanted to speak with me if I had a few minutes. I said, "Sure," and he led me over to a corner of the club.

His wife, named Marie, was about thirty-five years old, brunette, and very good-looking. She was dressed totally in black leather and was carrying a riding crop—definitely a dominant!

Marie confirmed this when she told me that she had been a professional dominatrix for several years. "I love being dominant over men," she said, "and I particularly like younger, strong men who can really take it."

"So what do you want with me?" I thought to myself.

She told me. "I'm truly dominant," she explained. "I don't do it just for the money. I love making a man my total slave." Then she took a deep breath. "But somewhere deep inside me I've always had this secret itch to see what it would be like to be a slave. To commit myself totally to a really dominant man; to be helpless, to be whipped, and to be used for his pleasure in any way he wanted to use me— just like I use my slaves."

Then she looked me straight in the eye. "I've never done it," she said, "because I've never met a man who excited me and who I thought would be strong enough to really dominate me as completely as I dominate my slaves." She reached out, took my hand, and kissed it. "Now I have," she said, "and I would be honored to be your slave for a night."

Three weeks later, Marie's husband brought her to my apartment. She was blindfolded, her hands were handcuffed behind her, and she was completely naked under her raincoat. As soon as I had opened the door, her husband pushed her inside. "I'll be back to get her in the morning," he said.

Marie got exactly what she was looking for, and we both had a very long and very exciting evening.

And ever since, she has come back once a year to scratch that same itch.

DIERDRE

I had been asked to put on a special S/M "demonstration" at the newly opened "Club O" in New York, and I'd picked a very special slave for the occasion. Her name was Dierdre. She was in her thirties but still had an almost perfect body. Even more important, she was genuinely submissive, could accept quite severe levels of discipline, and, best of all, had a well-developed sense of the theatrical.

There was a pretty big crowd, since Jill and Lily, the two ladies who ran "Club O," had advertised the event. At the appropriate moment, Jill turned off the music and introduced me. I began by explaining to the gathering my feelings about S/M, with particular emphasis on my strong feelings that while slaves may be submissive, they are still equals, and how much pleasure it gave me for an "equal" to give herself to me.

I then moved to the main stage, introduced Dierdre, and, as I talked some more, I had her slowly strip. She was then chained, her arms over her head, and I began whipping her very slowly. I continued the whipping for perhaps twenty minutes, carefully building the severity until, at the end, my cat-o'-nine-tails was cutting into Dierdre's naked back with considerable force and her body was jerking violently in reaction to each lash.

Finally I stopped and untied Dierdre, who promptly knelt and kissed my feet and my whip before I ordered her to move to a smaller platform in the center of the room where, as a finale, I planned to put needles into both her breasts before suspending her totally from the chains in the ceiling for a final whipping.

Standing on a small portable platform, Dierdre was chained, and I carefully inserted two very fine needles into each of her breasts. Then, while she was still standing on the riser, I whipped her back with a special long, single-strand, black leather whip. The effect on the crowd watching this lovely and totally obedient slave submitting to this new whipping, combined with the piercing of her breasts, was almost electric.

As a finale I had planned to remove the needles, suspend Dierdre totally, and finish by using that same whip on the front of her body. When I was ready, I turned her so that her back was to the audience and carefully began to remove the needles.

And then it happened! As one of the needles was removed, a tiny but steady trickle of blood began running down Dierdre's right breast. I hadn't planned it. I hadn't even expected it. I knew Dierdre wasn't hurt but I was instantly worried about the emotional effect on her. As it turned out, I was worried for no reason.

Dierdre looked down, saw the blood, and instantly looked up at me. And then, despite the pain of the whipping she had already endured and the knowledge that she was about to be totally suspended and whipped across her breasts, she flashed me a quick grin that the audience couldn't see. "Oh, wow!" she whispered. "Is that beautiful! Make the most of it!"

My reaction was immediate. With one hand I smeared the blood across Dierdre's breasts. Then, pulling the riser from under her so that she was hanging by her wrists, I quickly whipped her twice across the breasts. Then I turned her suspended body to face the audience.

There was a gasp that cut through the entire room. What they saw was a naked girl hanging by her wrists. She had just been whipped across the breasts, which were smeared with blood, and there was a slow trickle of blood running across both breasts and down onto her belly. And as I proceeded to lash Dierdre, the whip picked up drops of blood so that soon her breasts and belly were striped with the marks of the whip, each one outlined with the crimson of her blood.

After giving Dierdre a total of twenty lashes, I put the platform back and unchained her wrists. She fell against me and her blood ran onto my chest. Then she hugged me and kissed me before finally turning to the audience and declaring in a proud voice, "I love this Master!"

The place went wild, and afterward, as Dierdre and I walked slowly through the crowd, I saw that some of the spectators were actually crying.

DONNA

Donna was, and is, a totally straight girlfriend and not involved in the S/M scene in any way. But on our second date I told her about my involvement in the scene. One reason for doing this was that I wanted to stop by the Eulenspiegel Society—a New York City S/M discussion group—to talk to someone for a minute, and I asked Donna if she wanted to come along.

She did, and when we got there, she was fascinated by the crowd and the speaker. She'd never known the "scene" was actually so well established and organized.

After I had talked to my friend for a few minutes, Donna and I stood at the back of the room. Suddenly I noticed a very tall young man standing near us, obviously wanting to speak to me. He caught my eye and I nodded, and he said, "Excuse me, Sir, but aren't you from Chicago?"

I said that I was, and at the same time I noticed that Donna was listening closely. Maybe having this huge guy call me "Sir" had caught her attention. At any rate, the man next asked if my name was Sir John Q___, and again I said yes.

Smiling, he reached out to shake my hand and then said, "Oh, I thought so! I saw you with your slave at the 'Club O' two years ago, and it was so beautiful I've dreamed about it ever since!"

He shook my hand again and walked away; I turned to see Donna staring at me. "Jesus Christ!" she said.

"What does that mean?" I asked.

"You weren't kidding, were you?"

"No," I told her, "I wasn't kidding at all."

Donna grinned, took my arm, and pulled me toward the door. "Come on, Sir John," she said. "I've never had a Master buy me a drink, but tonight's the night!"

ALLISON

An early "Golden Moment" was provided by one of the most remarkable women I have ever met.

Her name is Allison, and she had always been a total "dominant" in the S/M scene. But over the years, we became close friends and then devoted lovers. Finally, despite her genuinely dominant nature, Allison made the decision to "give" herself to me.

It was the most precious gift that Allison could possibly offer me but, as she told me, it was the only way she felt she could properly express the depth of her love. And to "commemorate" that gift, she wrote me a very, very special letter.

John:

I have something to say to you that is so important and so special that I feel I must write it down to make sure that I say it exactly right.

I have always known that I am a very special person. I am intelligent. I am attractive. I am strong-willed. In short, I am superior.

That is why all of my adult life I have been what people call a dominant female. And I am dominant in all ways. Men have always recognized this and they have submitted to me. They have submitted intellectually; they have submitted emotionally; they have submitted sexually; and they have submitted physically, including submitting to my whip. They submit for one reason. I am stronger than they are, and I am better than they are.

But all of my life I have also hoped to meet just one man who was my equal. A man who not only could appreciate what and who I am, but who could also match my strength and superiority with his own equal strength and superiority.

I have finally found such a man. His name is John Q____. And I am in love with him.

I know who you are, John, and I know what you are. You are a complete man. You are a true dominant. And you are the only total Master I have ever met.

But what is most important is that just as I have recognized you as my equal, you have recognized me as yours.

That is why I love you, and because I love you, I am going to do something I have never done before and will never do again. I hereby give myself to you. Totally. Not *as a slave.* Not *as a submissive. Instead, I give myself to you as an* equal *who, of her own free will, chooses to be your* Lady.

My love is without reservation and so my gift is without reservation. I give you my mind and my body to use in any way you choose.

And because I know that you love taking pain from a woman's body, I know that your use of me will involve your whip. I want you to know that I am totally prepared to accept it.

I know my body gives you pleasure in all *ways. But I also know that one of the greatest sources of pleasure for you would be to inflict pain on my body. That body is now yours.*

I hate *pain. But I* love *you. And since I know that my pain will give you pleasure, then that is my gift to the one man in the world who deserves it.*

I give you my body—freely—and I invite you to use it for your pleasure. I love you, and so you are welcome to do things to me that no other man will ever do without killing me first. (Of course, you have the right to allow others to whip or use my body should that also give you pleasure. But in my mind that will still be you, and their bodies and their whips will simply be an extension of John Q＿＿'s will.)

I am yours. At any time you choose and in any place you choose, you may take me, strip me, chain me, whip me, torture me. I dedicate my body to your pleasure.

Take my pain as my gift of love. My body will writhe under your whip and my voice may scream, but my mind will glory in the pleasure that my pain gives to the man I love . . . and to the man who loves me.

The greater the pain the greater the gift, and I am determined to give you all that I am capable of giving. There are no *limits. So don't worry, John. Take your gift. Make my pain as great and as prolonged as you choose.*

And know that each time your whip bites into my body, along with the pain will come your own special way of saying that you love me just as I love you.

You deserve the best, John. I am *the best. And now the best is yours.*

Your Lady,

Allison

FRANCES

Finally, the "Pledge of Slavery" that my slave Frances asked me to draw up for her was perhaps the most special "Golden Moment" of all.

That pledge appears on the following page.

PLEDGE OF SLAVERY

I, frances _____, of my own free will and great desire, and based on absolute trust, do hereby give myself as a total slave to Sir John Q   and solmenly pledge the following:

. My name is frances.

. I am a slave.

. My Master is Sir John Q   and I belong to him solely and totally. I will never again ever refer to any other person by the title of "Master" or "Mistress".

. I will do for my Master absolutely anything he asks.

. My Master may do to or with me absolutely anything he desires.

. My Master, or anyone he chooses for his pleasure, may, in public or in private, whip or otherwise subject any part of my body to abuse in absolutely any manner, by absolutely any method, and with absolutely any implement my Master may choose.

. My Master, or anyone he invites for his pleasure, male or female, may, in public or in private, use my body for absolutely any sexual purpose whatsoever, and I will totally, willingly and actively cooperate in and respond to all such sexual activities.

. I pledge to my Master total devotion and instant, unquestioning obedience to any and every order he may give me, in public or in private. I acknowledge that if I should ever fail to provide such devotion or obedience, my Master will have the right to punish me in absolutely any way he deems appropriate, and I will humbly submit to that punishment no matter what or how severe that punishment may be.

. My Master and I recognize that I have given myself to him as a total slave of my own free choice and therefor, also of my own free choice, I may, at any time and in any place, end that slavery simply by kneeling and saying to him, "Master, I do not wish to be your slave any longer." However, I also fully understand that by making that statement I may totally and forever sever all relationships of any kind with Sir John Q

. I also fully understand that Sir John Q   has accepted me as his total slave of his own free choice. In recognition of that acceptance he will present me with his chain and lock and I will, with my own hands, place that chain around my neck and lock it there, knowing that only my Master holds the key. However, at any time and in any place, my Master may also dismiss me as his slave simply by ordering me to kneel, unlocking and removing his chain, and saying to me, "I do not wish to have you as my slave any longer."

In recognition and total acceptance of all of the above, with great pride, and in complete trust, I now give myself in total and absolute submission as a slave to my Master, Sir John Q   , and I make and sign this Pledge of Slavery, pierce my breast with a thorn from the rose my Master has given me to symbolize his respect and caring for me as his slave, and seal this pledge with my blood.

_____   10/29/85
        slave frances   Date

With great pride, and in recognition of her total trust in me, I hereby accept frances ____ as my total slave, I assume all responsibilities that go with that acceptance, and, as her Master, I sign this Pledge of Slavery and seal it with my blood.

_____   10/29/85
        Sir John Q   Date

16

Rose

It's going to be very easy to write about Rose because, for the most part, she has written her own chapter through a series of the most beautiful and exciting letters and notes a slave has ever written me. Even more important, those notes and letters provide the most complete and intelligent insight into the thoughts and motivations of a submissive that I have ever read.

It began while I was still living in Chicago. I had placed an advertisement in several S/M publications seeking a new slave and received numerous answers. One from a young lady in Indiana named Rose was so perfect that the rest seemed dull. It read:

My Dear Sir,

How can I possibly expain how very special I am and how very different from all the other women who have written to you?

First, a few statistics. I am twenty-six years old, 5' 6", with long blonde hair, blue eyes, and a 117-lb. 34-24-35 body that is in great shape.

But I'm sure you've had many beautiful women before, so what makes me special? I hope it is my devoutly submissive nature. I want to give myself in total submission to just one very special man who will, in turn, appreciate how very special I am. Please understand that

I am not one of those women who are submissive because they have low self-esteem. I am proud of who and what I am, and I want a man who will in turn be proud of me. Proud of my intelligence, proud of my strong will, proud of my character, proud of my beauty. And, most important, proud of his ownership of such a woman.

My sexuality is based on submissiveness. I receive tremendous sexual pleasure from simply being taken and used for the sexual pleasure of a man in whatever way he chooses. Understand, this is selfish on my part. The fact that I can give such pleasure rewards me equally.

And it goes beyond sex. I want to be allowed to serve my man in every way. In private, with those who share our understanding of such a relationship, I would hope to be ordered to display my submissiveness in any way he chooses. To others, they will see only my love, respect, and total dedication to his pleasure.

Of course, there is a problem with the fact that I live in Indianapolis. But Indianapolis is not that far from Chicago, and I am willing to go more than halfway to make it work.

Please write to me and at least give me the chance to convince you in person how much pleasure I could add to your life. I promise you won't be disappointed.

Hopefully,

Rose C_____

We met, of course, three weeks later in a motel halfway between her home and mine, and Rose quickly proved that she had been totally honest. In person she was equally as open, honest, and intelligent as she had been in her letter. She was sincerely submissive. And she was breathtakingly beautiful. Rose stayed with me that night and I whipped her three separate times.

During the last whipping, while she was tied spread-eagled on the bed, Rose asked permission to speak. When I gave it, she said, "Sir, I've never been whipped this severely but I don't want you to stop. So I'd appreciate it if you would gag me so that I can't scream or beg."

I did as she asked.

After that meeting, I received the following letter.

My Dear Sir,

Just one meeting and you already own me!

I'll admit how terrified I was when we first met out by the pool. First, I was afraid of what might happen to me. But after talking with you for a while, I was even more afraid that you might not accept me. You had explained to me that you never accepted a new submissive without meeting her and "evaluating" her. I felt as if I was being interviewed for a job and I was so afraid that I might not measure up.

But then you invited me to dinner and my whole body trembled with joy and, by the time the motel door closed behind us later that night, I knew I had found the man I wanted and that I was committed.

Oh God, how special that night was! I had told you that I had been with a couple of other "dominant" men before, but never anyone like you. So sure of yourself, so strong, and so unafraid to take whatever pleasure you wanted from me. You also know that I had been whipped before but, again, never the way you whipped me. You whipped me so expertly and the pain was more than I had ever experienced before, but at the same time I never doubted that you that you really cared for me and that you also knew exactly how much I could take. And so, when I finally asked you to gag me, it was because I didn't want to have even the chance of begging you to stop or let me go.

Please understand, I am not a masochist. Pain is pain, and you certainly tested my ability to endure it. But along with the physical pain came the tremendous psychological pleasure of knowing that somehow that gift would be returned.

And I was so right! I lay there naked on the bed after my last whipping, my wrists still tied to the headboard, and then I felt your hands and your mouth and your tongue slowly exploring my body so gently, caressing the marks of your whip. And then you untied my ankles and I finally felt the wonderful hardness of your body as it slowly entered mine and I knew right then that there was absolutely nothing that I wouldn't do to keep that feeling a part of my life forever.

Thank you, Sir, for accepting me and for the most wonderful night of my life. I know I gave you pleasure, too, and I can only promise to learn how to give you more and more pleasure . . . more than any woman has ever given you.

Yours,

Rose

A week later, Rose spent two days with me in my Chicago apartment, and after she returned home she sent another note.

. . . I can't tell you how excited I was during the drive from Indianapolis to Chicago, knowing that for two whole days I was going to be totally owned by my wonderful new Master. I had no idea what you might do to me or with me . . . only that my Master owned me completely and would do anything he wanted to.

And when you finally tied me bent over the chair and took me from behind it drove me wild. I saw you coming to me and I saw your magnificently hard erection and I knew you were going to satisfy your body, but I also knew that I would be satisfied, too.

Master, I want you to use my body for your pleasure alone. That is a basic part of my submissive nature. But I assure you that by doing that you will fulfill me as well.

Yours,

Rose

Our relationship grew quickly in intensity. Rose's submission was total, and she just naturally fell into the "slave" role. Whenever we were together, she never performed even the simplest act without asking any permission. (I remember her once saying, "I'd like to be so totally dominated that my Master could tell me when to breathe.") Whenever I sat, Rose would kneel at my feet. She would not look me in the eye unless ordered to do so.

Rose submitted gladly and totally to quickly increasing levels of both physical discipline and sexual submission. The letter she sent after her next trip to Chicago commented on the discipline.

My Dear Sir John,

I am learning how important the whip is to you—more important than it was to any of the other men I used to let dominate me. But please understand that it makes no difference. I am your slave and yours to use in any way you choose.

I just want to learn as much about your needs and desires as I can as quickly as I can, because I am devoted to fulfilling them, just as you fulfill mine. And if that means more and more of the whip, well then, that's what I'm there for because my *needs and desires are to be a total slave.*

I do not need the whip, but as a slave I will gladly serve all of my Master's desires, completely apart from my own. And with such a Master as you, that service is by itself a source of such tremendous pride and pleasure for me, including the pride and pleasure of being able to give my Master more and more of my pain.

Yours,

Rose

And in a letter Rose wrote about her feelings regarding sexual submission, she said:

. . . I have often told you that the bottom line of my nature is sexual submission.

That is so much more than simply being tied to a bed and being fucked. Of course, that's great and I love orgasms as much as any woman. But knowing that you are doing it only *for the pleasure it gives* you *is even better than a orgasm.*

You have the right to use me sexually in any way you choose, and even the right to order me to serve others sexually. I want to know that while you may hope it gives me pleasure, too, I have no right to resist whether it pleases me or not. I want to know that you will do whatever you want just for yourself.

That doesn't lessen my pleasure from sex. Instead, it heightens it. As your slave, your pleasure is my only thought, but I am your slave because it also gives me such great pleasure.

In short, for me submission and sex are inseparable.

This is from another letter:

I always seem to be writing to you about my basic sexually submissive nature. Maybe the following fantasy, one of my very favorites and one that I have had for years, will give you a better idea of how deep these feelings are.

I have been taken by five men to serve their sexual pleasure. They are all young, large, strong, and very capable sexually. They strip me and tie me bent forward over a large padded sawhorse. My legs are spread wide and tied to the outside legs. It is not painful . . . they do not intend to whip me or cause me pain in any other way. They just want me to be helpless . . . with every part of my body available to them and without any possibility of my resistance.

They draw lots, and the first man comes to stand in front of me and orders me to suck his cock. I do so until it is hugely erect. Then he moves behind me and begins fucking my pussy while the second man orders me to suck his cock. It continues that way. When the first one comes inside my pussy, the second takes his place and I am now sucking the cock of the third man.

Finally each has had his turn, but it does not end. Instead, I am again ordered to use my mouth to "prepare" them, and when each one is again fully erect, he fucks me a second time, this time in my ass. It continues until they have all climaxed once more.

It is still not over. Again I am ordered to suck each man's cock until they have all had a third orgasm, and this time I swallow their sperm.

For hours, every orifice of my body has been used sexually by all five men. Each one has fucked me in my pussy, and then in my ass, and finally in my mouth. That use of my body has been solely for their sexual pleasure. . . .

But because of this selfish use of my body, and my knowledge that this use of me is only for their pleasure, I have lost count of the number of marvelous orgasms I have experienced.

Perhaps this disclosure, from still another letter, was the bluntest of all:

Beyond all else I am sexually submissive. My choice to be your slave is completely sexual in intent. I submit to your chains and your whips only for sexual pleasure. I will endure anything that leads to my finally being rendered helpless and then being fucked. And fucked. And FUCKED!

A few weeks later, Rose wrote to me about one of her fantasies. When she arrived at my Chicago apartment, she knelt and handed me an envelope. On the outside was written, "Master . . . a fantasy meant to come true." And inside there was a letter.

I have always had fantasies, but until I met you I never considered them to be anything else. But now that I know you, I also know that no matter how bizarre a fantasy may seem to me, you are totally capable of making it very real. That is why, until now, I have resisted telling them to you, but you are my Master and you have told me that it would please you to hear them. So here goes.

I am kneeling on the floor in front of you. You sip your wine and then reach out to caress my breasts. After a while you order me to strip to the waist and you slowly begin to torment my nipples, pulling and pinching and twisting them—harder and harder. The pain and the pleasure grow for me and when I finally cry out it is an expression not just of the pain but also of the intense pleasure it gives me. Then, when I am almost ready to beg, you stop, but then your fingers are replaced by your nipple clamps.

You then order me to strip completely, and when I have you pull me across your lap and begin my spanking. It goes on and on, harder and harder. Meanwhile, the fingers of your other hand are caressing my clit and exploring my very wet pussy.

You tell me that I will be spanked until I have an orgasm, and when your hand gets tired you begin using that hard leather paddle that I gave you for your birthday. I don't know how long this goes on but finally, although I am now crying freely, I experience a total, marvelous, incredibly great orgasm that completely blots out all the pain.

Then you chain me standing up with my arms stretched high over my head. You gag me and remove the nipple clamps and then my whipping begins. My fantasy does not include details of how long or how hard I am whipped, but I know that as long as it lasts I will see that wonderful look of pleasure in your eyes.

After my whipping you take me to the bedroom and tie me spread-eagled and face-up on the bed. I am still gagged and I am tied so tightly that I can hardly move.

And then you fist fuck me, and I have another incredible orgasm.

Finally, you remove the gag, untie me, and then retie me in a hog tie, my wrists tied tightly to my ankles behind my back. And then you kiss me goodnight and you leave, and I know that I will spend the night tied that way while my body remembers over and over again both the pain and the pleasure.

Your slave,

Rose

Rose was constant in her efforts to learn how to please me and also to explain how she felt. For example, on one particularly intense evening, she had "challenged" me to make her quit. She chose the tests, which included hanging her by her wrists; tormenting her nipples with a needle; and, finally, for the first time, "raping" her in her ass. After that evening, Rose wrote to me:

My Dearest Master,

Last night was the fulfillment of my dearest fantasy. Being tied bent forward over that chair and then feeling your wonderfully hard cock being slowly forced into my ass. It was right that I was helpless so that I could not possibly even hope to resist, even if it lasted all night. And now I am completely *yours. You have used every part of my body for your pleasure.*

And now you also know that I will never back down from a challenge, particularly one that I have suggested. You allowed me to choose how long I would hang by my wrists. I knew that the longest I had ever done that was about six minutes. That's why I chose ten minutes. The last two or three minutes were so very hard, but your slave is proud that she did not beg and I was rewarded by that wonderful look of surprise and admiration on your face.

And then the needle in my nipple! I know it was me who chose that challenge but still I was so scared. And it hurt . . . oh, God, how it hurt! But again I was rewarded by that wonderful look on your face.

I want to see you again, as soon as you will allow me to, and now you know that I am totally capable of giving you pleasure in absolutely any way you choose. And I look forward to giving you that pleasure for the rest of your life.

Your slave,

Rose

Rose would also bring me "gifts." For example, after I had been away on a 2-week trip, Rose visited me in my Chicago apartment. Upon arriving she handed me an envelope, and then asked that I hang her by her wrists before opening it. I did so. Here's what her note said:

Dearest Master,

Thank you for allowing me to present this "welcome home" gift to you.

By the time you have finished reading this letter, I will be naked and gagged and will have been hanging by my wrists for three or four minutes. Now I would like you to put those very tight clamps on my nipples and then, using your fingers and/or vibrator, play with me until I have an orgasm. That will be my gift to myself.

Now for my gift to you. No matter how long it takes me to have an orgasm, I want you to whip me for the same length of time. Of course, I don't know if I will even be able to have an orgasm while hanging this way or how long it might take. I may be here for a very long time. That is why the gag is important. I don't want to have any chance of taking back my gift.

Finally, after my whipping, I beg the reward of having you take me down and then feeling your cock in my mouth and then in my pussy and finally in my ass until you climax.

Welcome home, Master. I hope this gift pleases you.

Your slave,

Rose

In September, Rose and I spent four and a half days together, two of which were spent at a special annual outing of the New York "S/M Couples Club" which was held at a private camp in the Poconos. Some fifty couples from all over the country attended, and it was a lot of fun. Afterward, Rose wrote:

My Dearest Master,

I once wrote you that I would prefer a life of submission twenty-four hours a day, seven days a week. The four days I just spent with you are proof that that desire is so right for me.

I was your total slave every minute, and it was so wonderful to be able to display my submission to you to people who share our world. I never grew tired or bored with your domination of me. Instead, I wanted it to last forever, and when I was forced to return to my other world I was sad.

I am in no way degraded by being your slave. Instead, I glory in it, and I loved being able to show off my submissive status. I remem-

ber hanging naked from the beams in the dining hall while you ate breakfast Saturday morning and seeing the looks of admiration on the faces of all the others and knowing that I am the luckiest slave in the world because I belong to Sir John Q____. (And I know that many of the other slaves were so jealous!)

And then that night when you invited other masters to whip me and use me sexually in any way they chose. To me, that was the essence of S/M . . . a Master so completely sure of his ownership of his slave and of her devotion to him that he feels no insecurity at all in lending her to others.

And finally you took me in front of the fireplace, bent me over the bench, and fucked me so roughly in my ass while the others watched. And I will never forget that while you were doing that, you grabbed my hair and pulled my head back and growled so only I could hear, "I will never let you go, slave. Never. And if you ever try to leave me, I will beat you within an inch of your life!"

To me, that is what S/M is all about.

Your eternally grateful slave,

Rose

The next month, Rose wrote me the most important letter of all.

Dearest Master,

What follows has always been my favorite fantasy, but I never dreamed that it could ever come true. Now your slave begs you to make it come true.

We have talked many times of my desire to have rings put in my nipples and have your initials branded on the inside of my thigh. You have explained that those acts are so permanent that we should wait until I am completely sure.

Master, I am sure. And here is my fantasy.

You have arranged to have me taken to a secluded, private home somewhere out in the country, and you have invited all your friends to witness this supreme test of my submission to my chosen Master and my formal initiation as your slave. Two servants take me to a private room where I am stripped, bathed, and then led into a huge

*living room. I notice that all the guests are dressed in semiformal attire
—the men in suits and ties and the women in cocktail dresses.*

*All the guests are standing except for you and a beautiful older
woman. You two are seated at one end of the living room in large
comfortable armchairs. Very quickly I am chained standing in the middle
of the room, my ankles secured to rings set in the floor and my arms
stretched high above my head.*

*The woman next to you rises and approaches me. At first she says
nothing, but then her hands reach out and she begins to stroke my
body, paying particular attention to my breasts and ass and belly and
then finally inserting three fingers into my now soaking wet pussy.*

*Then she stands back and addresses me for the first time. "Slave
rose," she says. "You have agreed to endure a test of your submission
to Sir John Q_____. If you pass this test, you will then be formally
initiated into that role as his slave. I warn you now that both the test
and the initiation will be very difficult. Consequently, you now have
one final chance to change your mind. If you do, you will be released
and be allowed to leave. But if you agree, you will not be allowed
to change your mind. Now, tell me your decision.*

*I raise my head for the first time and look you in the eyes. And
then I speak. "Please proceed," is all I say.*

*It begins with a whipping. One of the servants uses a single-strand
leather whip and begins whipping me very slowly. At first the lashes
are not too hard, but slowly they become harder and harder, causing
me to wince and cry out softly as my entire body is slowly covered
by the marks of the whip. I don't know how long it goes on but suddenly,
while the whipping continues, I see a young woman, perhaps twenty
years old, enter the room. She, too, is naked and she is superbly beautiful—her body strong and tight, her belly flat, her perfectly formed
breasts high and very firm—and she has long, straight blonde hair that
hangs almost to her waist.*

*She crosses the room and kneels before you. She kisses your hand
and then carefully opens your pants, takes out your cock, and lowers
her head to it. And as she sucks your cock, you stroke her hair and
look at me. The whipping continues and I understand that I am to
experience watching you receive pleasure while I endure pain, also for
your pleasure. Part of me is so jealous. She is so beautiful and I know
how expert her mouth must be. But I also know that this is part of*

my test and I am so proud to have the chance to prove my total submission to my Master's pleasure.

The whipping continues. Every part of my body is now covered by the marks of the lashes. The pain grows and grows until I am afraid that I might faint, but suddenly your back arches and I know you have had an orgasm. Then you lift one finger and the whipping stops.

The blonde leaves the room and I am unchained, but almost immediately the two servants bring in a large, wide, cushioned bench and place it in the middle of the room. They lay me down on the bench face up, and then tie my wrists and ankles to the corners. Another stranger enters the room. He is a very large black man, maybe thirty years old and very muscular. He is wearing only a black silk robe.

He walks over the the bench where I am tied, naked and helpless. Slowly he walks around the bench, studying my nude body. Finally he stops and bends over. One hand cups my breast, still covered by the vivid marks left by the whip. He pinches my nipple and I wince, and then he says, "It is going to be such a great pleasure to violate you."

A table is wheeled in and on it are displayed a variety of dildos of all sizes. The man starts with a small one, carefully greasing it before inserting it into my pussy. He slowly moves it in and out, and at first I experience pleasure. But then he proceeds to use larger and larger dildos until finally I feel as if something must tear. When he has finished "fucking" me with the largest dildo, he stops but leaves the dildo inside of me. And then I see him carefully greasing his hand.

The large dildo is removed and then I feel his hand moving into me. One finger, two fingers, three, four, and finally, with a sudden thrust, his entire hand is inside me. His fingers curl into a fist and he forces it deeper and deeper until almost half his forearm is inside my body. Then he begins to fist fuck me, pulling his fist almost all the way out of my pussy and then ramming it back in as far as it will go, over and over again.

At last he removes his fist and I am again untied, but almost immediately I find myself being retied, this time bent forward over a padded sawhorse, my ankles tied wide to the legs on one side and my wrists to the legs on the other side. The dildo ritual begins again, but this time they are inserted in my ass, and I feel myself being stretched farther and farther. Finally a huge dildo, two or three inches thick and at least ten inches long, is inserted into my ass and left there. And then the man removes his robe and I see that his fully erect cock is at least as large as the dildo still inside me.

The dildo is removed and instantly replaced by his cock. It feels even larger than the dildo and as he begins to fuck me in the ass, I hear him speak again. "I'm going to make this last a very long time," he says. It does, for almost half an hour.

Finally I am removed from the sawhorse and the servants take me to a private bathroom where I am allowed to bathe and freshen myself. Perhaps an hour later I am taken back to the living room and again tied face up on the padded bench, but this time so tightly that I can barely move a muscle. You approach me and for the first time I hear you speak.

"You are wonderful, slave," you say, "and I am so very, very proud of you. You have passed the tests superbly and now I am going to make you mine forever."

Another table is wheeled in and on it I see the needles. I know that at last my dream is about to come true, and I hope the pain is great. Slowly you pass a needle through my right nipple, and I gasp but manage not to scream. You leave that first needle there and pierce the other nipple. Then beautiful gold rings replace the needles, and I see that each one is fitted with a delicate gold chain with a tiny round pendant. On one is engraved the initial "J" and on the other the initial "Q."

But the ceremony is not over yet. Still another table is wheeled in and I see that it holds a small, white-hot branding iron bearing those same initials. "I love you, slave," you say, and I respond, "I love you, too, Master."

And then you lift the branding iron and begin to lower it to the quivering flesh on my right thigh.

Please know, Master, that I really want this. Once I am wearing your rings and bearing your brand you will own me totally. You will have the right to order me to be with you whenever you want; the right to order me to leave my job and move to Chicago; the right to use my body for your pleasure in any way you choose, twenty-four hours a day; and even the right to give me to whomever you choose, allowing them to use your slave for their pleasure, just because it pleases you to do that.

Please, *Master, let this fantasy come true.*

Your devoted slave,

Rose

This "fantasy" started us on the most exciting S/M adventure of all. In short, Rose wanted to have her Master pierce her nipples and have gold rings put in them. But, to her mind, that also meant that she would belong *totally* to that Master, living with him in a life of full-time, 24-hour-a-day submission. Obviously, I was not ready for that, but I was completely willing to commit to her totally for every minute of that part of my life that was involved with the "scene."

And so plans were begun. I was determined to do the piercing myself, so I flew out to Los Angeles and personally visited a store called "The Gauntlet." This store specializes in piercing equipment and jewelry, and the people there were tremendously helpful. I bought two beautiful gold rings. I also bought special piercing needles, piercing forceps, and a book carefully explaining in detail how piercings should be done.

I also began making the arrangements for the "initiation." Anne P_____ is a beautiful, experienced, and thoroughly delightful "dominatrix," and it pleased me tremendously when Anne told me how "honored" she was by my request to hold the ceremony in the huge, fully equipped "discipline room" that she then maintained on the third floor of her New Jersey home.

Anne also arranged to invite "Sir Michael," a well-known dominant, to the ceremony. Since he had performed dozens of piercings, Anne felt he would be helpful. She was very right.

The date selected by Rose and me was February 14 . . . Valentine's Day. As I've already tried to make clear, the piercing of Rose's nipples was something far, far beyond a normal S/M scene. Instead, it was a symbol of exactly what we meant to each other; since love played an important part in our relationship, it seemed appropriate that we commit ourselves to each other on that special day.

With the expert help of Anne's head slave, Viola, an elaborate party had been planned. Hors d'oeuvres, caviar, and champagne had been ordered, and Viola had even written and mailed to each guest a special letter designed to make sure the "tone" of the party was maintained in accordance with the plans. The letter read:

Dear Friend:

You recently received an invitation to a very special affair—the formal testing, initiation, and nipple-piercing of Master John Q____'s slave, rose. Despite the fact that rose will be very severely tested by several Mistresses and Masters, it is intended for this to be an absolutely beautiful and truly memorable ceremony.

It will be attended by invitation only, *and each invitation will admit just one couple, unless specifically arranged otherwise* in advance.

Master John has requested that you dress as you would to attend a "semi-formal" Sunday afternoon cocktail party. Jackets and ties are preferred for the men, and dresses or suits for the ladies. (No S/M costumes, please.*)*

Please be prompt. Because of the very special nature of the ceremony, it will not be possible to admit anyone after it has begun. The ceremony has been scheduled to begin at 3:00 P.M. sharp.

Several dominants will be invited to participate in the ceremony, helping to "test" slave rose. If you are asked, and if you agree, we ask that you please allow Mistress Anne to direct your participation, as Master John has asked that Mistress Anne direct the overall ceremony.

As those of you who were at the gathering in the Poconos last September already know, slave rose as an absolutely beautiful young lady. The careful planning of the ceremony in which her submission will be tested, combined with the decor of the overall affair, assures that this will be an S/M event of taste and drama and sensitivity and importance that will never be forgotten.

We hope that you will be able to honour us with your attendance. Please RSVP as soon as possible.

Thank you.

viola
head of household staff
Mistress Anne P____'s Residence

Rose and I arrived at noon, and she was turned over to a lovely little submissive, Jane, who had been selected to act as Rose's "attendant." Jane took Rose up to a separate suite that connected to the "discipline room," and stayed with her while Rose bathed and got herself ready for her ordeal.

The guests, who began arriving at two o'clock, were served champagne in the main floor living room. Then, promptly at 3:00, they were all invited to gather on the third floor; after Anne had introduced the several prominent dominants and dominatrixes who had agreed to participate, the ceremony began.

I led Rose into the room, dressed only in a full-length black negligee. Upon my signaled command, she stepped up on the low platform "stage" and knelt obediently. After introducing Rose, I turned the proceedings over to Anne, who began by having Rose repeat the standard "slave litany" that my slaves have always been taught.

Anne: "What is your name?"

Rose: "My name is Rose."

Anne: "What are you?"

Rose: "I am a slave."

Anne: "Who is your Master?"

Rose: "My Master is Sir John Q_____.

Anne. "What can your Master do to or with you?"

Rose: "Anything he desires."

Anne: "What will you do for your Master?"

Rose: "Anything that he asks."

Anne: "What is your only purpose in life as a slave?"

Rose: "My only purpose is to serve my Master's pleasure in any way he chooses."

Then, in a prelude "lifted" from Rose's fantasy, Anne explained to her that her Master had arranged for her to be tested to prove the sincerity of those vows. Anne told Rose that she would have to undergo two tests. The first would be a test of her physical submission, during which she would be severely disciplined. The second would be a test of her sexual submission. Finally, Anne explained that, if she wanted to, Rose could choose to leave right then, but that if she stayed, she would not be allowed to change her mind.

In a very quiet voice, Rose said, "I accept the test." Anne ordered Rose to stand and strip, and then she was immediately chained standing in a spread-eagled position. Just before the first test began, Anne explained to Rose that while she would be permitted to scream, her Master did not expect her to beg for mercy.

And then the first test began. Six different Masters and Mistresses had been selected to take part. Each one tried in turn to force Rose to "break," either by calling them "Master" or "Mistress," which I had expressly forbidden her ever to do; or to look them in the eye, which was also forbidden; or to ask them to stop. Each dominant delivered five strokes of his or her own selected whip or riding crop. Although relatively brief, each individual whipping was quite severe, but Rose was magnificent. Repeatedly she was forced to cry out as the whips cut into her body, but as each new dominant stepped up and said, "Call me 'Master,' Rose," Rose would whisper, "I can't, sir. My Master won't allow it."

The last dominant to whip Rose was Diane, a beautiful young lady with long blonde hair falling below her waist. For this occasion she was dressed in a stunning full-length black gown. I had asked her to use my cat-o'-nine tails, and she had secretly been limited to twenty-five lashes. But she told Rose that there were *no* limits and that she was going to whip her until she called her "Mistress," no matter how long it took. Almost as if she were stalking her prey, Diane walked slowly around and around Rose's spread-eagled form. "Call me Mistress!" she would order, as the cat would whistle through the air and Rose would cry out yet again when the nine braided leather strands bit into her body. "Call me Mistress, damn it!" Diane ordered. "I can't," Rose whispered, and the whip would whistle again. There was dead silence in the room as the guests, almost holding their breaths, waited to see if Rose would break.

After the twenty-fifth stroke, Diane stood back and handed the cat to Anne, who announced that Rose had passed the first test. But it wasn't quite over. That morning Rose had presented me with a Valentine card, and on it was written the following note:

My Dearest Master,

Although I do not know exactly what will be done to me today, I do remember my special fantasy and I would like to beg for one change. No matter how long or how hard I am whipped by others, I ask to have the marks of your whip the last ones left on my body.

Your total slave,

rose

Rose had taken a far more severe whipping than she had ever expected, and so before I began I went to her, stroked her hair and her body, and quietly asked her if she still meant what she had said in her note. "Yes, Sir," she whispered.

I didn't make it easy for her. First I ordered that the ropes holding Rose's arms be raised and the platform removed so that she would be completely suspended. Then I took a special long, single-strand, black leather "snake" whip and began this final part of Rose's first test. Originally I had intended to deliver a total of ten lashes. Properly used, this whip concentrates all its bite into one little area. It doesn't cut. It doesn't bruise. But the pain is quite severe.

Rose remained silent during the first three lashes, trying, I think, to show me just one more time how magnificently gutsy she is. But on the fourth lash she screamed and she continued to scream each time the "snake" bit her. I stopped after seven lashes.

The platform was replaced, Rose's body was lowered, and her arms and legs unchained. I hugged her once, kissed her gently, and then turned her over to Anne again for the second test.

Again, this test had been suggested by Rose's fantasy. Still naked, she was ordered to kneel. From among the guests stepped Master Jack, a tall, powerful, black dominant well known not only in New York but throughout the country. True to his usual form, Master Jack was wearing studded leather cuffs and a black robe, and as he approached Rose the tension in the room grew even greater. First Jack ordered Rose to stroke his cock with her hands, and she obeyed. Once hard, he then ordered Rose to take his fully erect cock in her mouth. Since Jack has a much larger than average cock, I think even he was surprised when Rose used her practiced "deep-throat" technique to take all of it. Jack stroked Rose's hair gently while she sucked him, but suddenly he roughly pulled his cock from her mouth and ordered Rose bound over a whipping bench.

Then, as brutally as possible, Master Jack raped Rose's ass, pumping his cock into her so powerfully that finally two dominants had to step forward and hold the bench in place until Jack reached his roaring climax.

The tests were over. Rose was again untied and little Jane led her back to her private quarters to shower and rest herself for the finale. Meanwhile, the guests went back down to the main floor for more champagne and hors d'oeuvres.

An hour later, the guests were reassembled in the "discipline room." Rose, this time wearing a pure white negligee, was brought back and chained to a massive wooden "X" cross that had been moved to the center of the room during the intermission.

The piercing began.

Before the ceremony Rose and I had discussed techniques and the fact that various methods could be used to considerably lessen or even eliminate the pain. Rose had rejected them all. True to her fantasy, she wanted to experience the full measure of pain. Sir Michael used the forceps to hold Rose's left nipple securely while I took one of the sterilized piercing needles and began.

It was one of the hardest things I've ever done in my life! Despite the special needles, extra sharp and lubricated, it took every bit of my strength and perhaps as long as twenty seconds to put the needle through Rose's nipple. The pain was absolutely excruciating, and Rose screamed the entire time. But despite the fact that her arms were only loosely chained over her head to the cross, she never moved a muscle!

Thank God Michael was there! I had intended not only to pierce Rose's nipples but also to put the gold rings in place; but by the time the needle was through that first nipple, my hand was shaking so badly that I asked Michael to put the ring in for me. This he did, quickly and with little additional pain to Rose. We gave Rose a few minutes to recover, and then we repeated the procedure on the right nipple.

It seemed to me that the entire procedure took forever. In reality, it only lasted about four minutes. But with the possible exception of the time I spent with Margot in Montreal, I have never, ever done anything that caused a slave such pain. More than that, never have I ever seen a slave with more love, commitment, and just plain guts than my Rose showed that afternoon.

It was over. Rose was unchained and presented with a dozen roses. The guests all applauded and, one by one, stepped forward to hug and kiss her. Then Rose went back to her quarters to wash her face and compose herself, and later she joined all of us for champagne.

That night, believe it or not, Rose and I went to the famous Hellfire Club in New York. Rose was wearing a gold lamé jump suit, opened to the waist to proudly exhibit her beautiful breasts with their new gold rings. She was smiling and happy and so very proud!

There is one postscript. A few days after the ceremony, Rose wrote a "thank you" note to Sir Michael. The following is a quote from that note:

. . . I am so happy and proud to be wearing my Master's rings. Although the pain was more severe than anything I have ever experienced before, you should know that my Master did explain to me that there were ways to almost eliminate the pain. I rejected them. I wanted it done just the way it was.

My thanks again.

Sir John Q_____'s slave,

rose

17

Beth
(An Open Letter to a Novice Submissive)

I had run an advertisement hoping to find a new submissive. I received several responses, one in particular from a young lady named Beth. Beth acknowledged that she was a total "novice" and had never actually had any S/M experiences; but she also said that she had, for several years, fantasized about being submissive, and thought that perhaps it was time for her to move from fantasy to reality. Before making that move, however, she asked if I would please write to her and answer some of the questions she had always wanted answered but had never had the nerve to ask anyone.

Beth's letter was so honest and sincere that I wound up writing her a long, long letter in which I tried, as best I could, to explain the "scene" as I saw it, what it meant to me, and what it might add to her life. That letter follows. I hope that for any other "novice submissives" who may read this book, it will provide some answers as well.

Dear Beth,

Thank you for answering my advertisement. It is rare, in my experience, for a "novice" (as you call yourself) to ever write such an open and honest letter as yours, and for that reason I'm going to try as hard as I can to answer it with equal openness and honesty.

To begin with, I'll respond to the comments you made about what kind of a man I might be. Your analysis is correct. I am not a man looking to "expand his stable." That would be a simple thing to do, but things that are simple hold no attraction for me.

You also say that you think I am a man of intelligence. You indicate that this is an important criterion for you. Well, it is an equally important criterion for me in my search for a submissive companion.

Any second-rate "Master" can, presumably, find and "dominate" one of the run-of-the-mill dull and abject "slaves" that so many of those self-proclaimed Masters seem to attract.

That kind of submissive doesn't interest me.

Anyone can have a "commoner" for a slave.

I require a queen!

I want someone of intelligence and breeding and wit and conviction so that when I become her Master, I can take pride in the fact that such a woman has chosen to devote her entire being to the satisfaction and fulfillment of my desires.

Just as she, in turn, can take pride that such a man has chosen her, above all others, to provide that fulfillment.

As for your questions about what motivates a "Master" and what might happen to you should you choose to actually give yourself to such a man, that's going to take much longer to answer.

For openers, should you decide that you may actually be a true submissive, and find the courage and commitment to put yourself in the hands of a true Master, you should know that at that precise moment your option to make choices will end. He will do what he wants to do, completely apart from your preconceived ideas.

I am not necessarily referring to physical discipline, and I am most definitely not referring to the extremes of physical discipline. There are always limits, and the true Master knows what they are. He also knows that those limits are different for every slave. But he also knows that, regardless of those individually determined limits, every slave should at least once be forced to go one small step beyond what she believes she can endure.

A Master should do what pleases him. The secret is to know the slave well enough so that while pleasing himself, he also provides her with fulfillment. But he should also once in a while take his slave— even if only for brief moments—slightly beyond her own self-conceived limits. But in doing so, he must take care not to really *hurt her.*

In short, a slave should, once in a while, be forced to beg—to plead, "Oh, God, please stop!" But after every session, a slave should also, if only just to herself, always say, "Oh, God, I want him to have me again!"

As I said, it doesn't have to be physical discipline. If you are lucky, you may someday find a Master who is also an expert at sensual "torture." If you have never experienced this, you may not believe it, but a Master who knows the art, and who is smart enough to learn what kind of a woman you are, will be able to "torture" you without hurting you at all!

The human body can voluntarily withstand only a certain level of sensual pleasure or sensation. That is why a man, when he has an orgasm, usually stops moving, because he just can't stand the sensation of having the tip of his penis stimulated while he is coming. That's also why a woman who has a true, full orgasm also usually stops moving, or arches her back and pulls her body taut, or fights or cries out or curls into a ball.

It *is* not *that it hurts.* It is just that the pleasure is unbearable!

But suppose you were tied and exposed and helpless. And suppose that your Master knew you well enough to be able to regularly bring you to full orgasm. And then suppose your Master did that and then kept you there—right at the peak—for perhaps five minutes or ten or even twenty minutes!

Imagine being at the very peak of a full orgasm that didn't stop!

Imagine straining at your bonds and screaming and pleading and begging for him to stop, and imagine him being good enough and strong enough to ignore your screams and to keep that sensual "torture" going on and on, because it pleases him to hear you scream and beg, and so he just keeps it going—not until you *beg him to stop but until* he *chooses to,* for himself.

This same principle is true of actual physical discipline, for those Master/slave relationships where true discipline is involved. Suppose that a slave could, without being bound, voluntarily withstand thirty lashes of a whip across her back. But then suppose she is bound, arms stretched high overhead, her body naked and helpless, and her Master begins her "test." And because she is proud, and because she wants to provide her Master with as much pleasure as possible, she does not actually "break" until after forty lashes, but then she begs him to stop.

If he is a true Master, and if it really brings him pleasure to continue, he should not stop. *Perhaps he will continue for another five lashes— or maybe ten, depending on his pleasure, of course, but also based on the knowledge he has, through experience, of just how much his slave can really endure, not simply what her body tells her she can endure. There is a difference.*

If the Master is wise and has been accurate in his assessment of his slave's true stamina, the slave will realize that she actually did endure it after all. Even more important, she will be proud that she was able to provide her Master with that additional pleasure, and the next time perhaps she won't begin to beg until after fifty lashes.

But of course her Master may not stop then, either!

It suddenly occurs to me that so far I haven't said anything about "sex." Probably that's because it is so obvious and so natural to me. But if you are, as you say, a "novice," it may not be at all obvious to you. So let me explain. To begin with, S/M is the most exciting form of sexual foreplay I have ever experienced, and I have learned that this is true for women as well. Every "Master/slave" relationship should be based on a profound and deeply satisfying sexual relationship. Every meeting should include (and usually conclude with) some form of sexual activity that is satisfying to both. But that, of course, is generally true of every deep male/female relationship. So what makes this any different?

The difference lies in the submission of one and the dominance of the other. That, of course, is what your own fantasies have been based on. In effect, you say you have dreamed of "submitting" yourself to a man, allowing yourself to be rendered helpless, so that he can "rape" you. And that act of submission, you say, would enhance the excitement and pleasure you would derive from the sex act. (Indeed, the truth may be that this is the only way that you would be able to derive real pleasure from sex.)

But if this is as far as you've gone in your fantasies, you may well be asking yourself, "What is all the rest about? Why does he talk about prolonged sexual teasing and torment? And what about real discipline . . . actual pain, even if only at a very minor threshold level? Would a Master really whip me?"

I have no idea, but the simple fact is that all these things, carefully selected and based on each partner's individual reaction, can be part of what becomes a much greater and much more rewarding and much more fulfilling sexual relationship. Sex, without some form of mutual love or deep feeling, is of little meaning and that, in turn, requires each partner to try to give the other as much pleasure as possible. For a submissive, that means "giving" herself to her Master, for his pleasure. *The total submission of her mind and body are her gifts to him, for him to do with as he chooses, and he takes great pleasure in that gift.*

Every Master is different, of course, so I can speak only for myself. I take tremendous pleasure in imposing my dominance and will upon a submissive female, both mentally and physically. I love using both her mind and her body to demonstrate my power over her. I love making her think and feel things she has never felt before. I love forcing her to experience the furthest extremes of sensual and physical sensations. I love, finally, making her beg me to stop either the pleasure or the pain.

Best of all, I love watching her face and her expression as she realizes that, despite her pleas, I am not *going to stop . . . at least not right at that minute. And, finally, I love watching her recognize my dominance over her, and then watching her resign her mind and her body to accept the previously unacceptable . . .* all for my pleasure!

Through all of this, and governing all of this, is the overriding "love" that I feel for her and, in turn, it is her knowledge that I do care for her very deeply, and the trust that that knowledge gives her, that allows her to make me that marvelous gift of her mind and body.

But what about the submissive one? What pleasure does she *get? Again, each is different, but there are at least some common denominators. First, a "slave" must both deeply trust and deeply care for her Master. She should truly want to give him pleasure. And so, for most slaves, the first pleasure is the very deep pleasure derived from the act of giving . . . a very profound pleasure because the gift she gives is also profound.*

She gives herself!

Second (although there are some exceptions), a submissive female usually derives tremendous intellectual, sensual, and, ultimately, sexual *pleasure from the experience, assuming, of course, that her Master is really gifted and sensitive and understanding. You have already alluded to this elemental source of pleasure in your letter, but I assure you that you have only scratched the surface. If we were to actually meet and find ourselves alone together, I would very likely teach you things about yourself you have never dreamed of . . . expose you to sources of pleasure of a kind and a level and an intensity you have never imagined!*

How? I don't have the faintest idea because I don't know you. But, given the chance, I would explore every part of your mind and body, and I would ultimately discover the keys to your deepest pleasures.

It may be strictly sensual. There may be certain special parts of your body that, properly stimulated, turn on all your sexual senses. Eventually I would find them and use them.

It may be just the bondage and helplessness itself, together with your ability to commit yourself to it. Most submissive women derive tremendous sexual pleasure simply from being bound. (Almost all of them become lubricated and ready for sexual intercourse while in bondage.)

You may find pleasure in pain. And if you do, it may be just a certain level of pain, or pain applied just to a certain part of your body. Many submissive people derive the most intense and exquisite sexual pleasure from the forced imposition of physical discipline, even to the point of orgasm.

You should also know that "discipline" doesn't mean simply the whip. (Although, indeed, that phrase "simply the whip" is totally misleading. There are literally hundreds of different kinds of whips, each capable of being used in a hundred different ways, so that in just this one "simple" area, there are an infinite variety of ways available to a knowledgeable Master to impose an equally infinite variety of torments.)

But there is so much, much more . . . endless means; endless targets; endless degrees. To a really imaginative and experienced Master, a marvelous and exquisite and almost limitless choice is available. But he must also have the sensitivity and the understanding and, yes, the love, to choose the right ones.

If he does, he will be successful in fulfilling his role as a Master. He will provide pleasure for himself, of his own choosing, but he will also provide his submissive partner with either extreme sexual pleasure or total psychological fulfillment or, often, both—depending on her own special nature and needs.

Then there is the whole area of submission without bondage. A true Master, using proper training, can teach a woman to be totally submissive without putting her in bondage. If you really have accepted a man as your Master, you should want to totally obey him without being "forced."

If he orders you to strip, you will strip. If he orders you to kneel, you will kneel. If he orders you to stand before him with your legs apart and your arms stretched high above your head, and not to move, you will do as he orders. And if, while you are standing there, he chooses to whip you, you still will not move. And if he orders you to count the lashes, you will count them for him.

And if he orders you to kneel, naked, next to his bed while he sleeps, and to remain there, instantly ready to serve him in any way should he awake, you will kneel there, silent and naked and ready, and you will stay *there. And if he does not awake until morning, you will* still *be there . . . still kneeling . . . still naked . . . still ready.*

But then a wise Master will order you to join him, and he will acknowledge the great pleasure your obedience has given him, and he will reward you with that special marvelous pleasure of your own that he knows so well how to give you.

That, Beth, is "what all the rest is about." A marvelously elaborate, infinitely varied, terribly exciting series of scenarios, carefully and lovingly selected and orchestrated by the Master to provide both himself and his submissive partner with the most exquisite and profound emotional and sexual pleasure—each scenario based on, taking advantage of, and dramatizing *the dominant nature of one and the submissive nature of the other.*

It is, of course, a tremendous challenge. First, there's the challenge to the submissive to accept and endure the torment of bondage and discipline by which her chosen Master tests her and through which he realizes the most profound pleasure. (A weak or sniveling "slave" provides little pleasure for a Master.) Of course, there are limits and, of course, they must be respected. But there will be those special times when, after being queried by her Master, the proud submissive will take as deep a breath as her chains will permit, look him in the eye, and in her own special way and words say, in effect, "I'm here for your pleasure. Please don't stop until you are totally satisfied."

That is a challenge of the body. But there is also the challenge of the mind and the spirit. After all, a man is usually physically stronger than a woman, so physical domination (in its rawest sense, at least) is easy.

But intellectually it's a different matter because in an ideal S/M relationship, both partners should be equal *in intellect, so that the dominant and submissive roles result from conviction and choice rather than imposition.*

But I also firmly believe that in addition to being physically dominant, a "Master"—while not intellectually superior—must also be intellectually dominant . . . *dominant by nature and spirit and* will . . . *choosing to dominate while the submissive chooses to understand and appreciate and ultimately submit to that will.*

That is a much more subtle and a far more difficult challenge.

I don't know what else I can tell you, Beth. I've probably told you too much already. But there is one more thing that you should know. I really am looking for "just one" very special woman who can, in turn, also appreciate how very special I am.

I want someone who, of her own free choice, is capable of giving herself to me with joy and pride.

Pride in herself; pride in her submissiveness; and pride in being "possessed" by a truly *experienced, imaginative, sensitive, and—yes— superior Master.*

I don't know if that someone is you.

But I will know very quickly if we should ever meet.

So will you.

But that decision is up to you.

The world for a truly *and* totally *and* actively *submissive woman can be one of incredible experiences and excitements and feelings and sensations and pleasures—pleasures which are intellectual and emotional and sexual.*

But you need two things. You need a Master who really knows how to lead you to these pleasures. And you need the courage to take the first step.

I can provide the first.

But you must provide the second.

I hope you do.

Sincerely,
Sir John Q———